STUDY GUIDE for

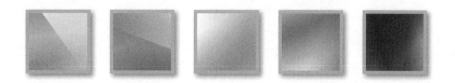

THE COMPLETE
MEDICAL ASSISTANT

STUDY GUIDE for

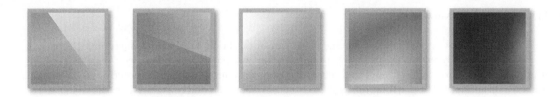

THE COMPLETE
MEDICAL
ASSISTANT

Janet R. Sesser, MS, BS, RMA (AMT)

Faculty Medical Assisting on Campus and Medical Billing and Coding Online
The Allen School of Health Sciences
Phoenix, Arizona

Deborah L. Westervelt, AS, RMA (AMT)

Registered Medical Assistant III/Clinical Supervisor
Washington University Orthopedics
St. Louis, Missouri

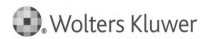 Wolters Kluwer

Philadelphia • Baltimore • New York • London
Buenos Aires • Hong Kong • Sydney • Tokyo

Acquisitions Editor: Jay Campbell
Senior Product Development Editor: Amy Millholen
Marketing Manager: Shauna Kelley
Senior Production Project Manager: Alicia Jackson
Design Coordinator: Teresa Mallon
Manufacturing Coordinator: Margie Orzech
Prepress Vendor: SPi Global

ISBN: 978-1-4963-8565-9

Preface

Welcome to the *Study Guide for The Complete Medical Assistant*. The Study Guide's exercises and activities align with the 2015 Core Curriculum for Medical Assistants established by the Medical Assisting Education Review Board (MAERB) of the American Association of Medical Assistants (AAMA). This guide also supports the 2017 Medical Assistant curriculum standards set forth by the Accrediting Bureau of Health Education Schools (ABHES). The Study Guide's exercises and activities are based on information presented in the textbook. The design of the exercises and activities meet various learning domains including cognitive, psychomotor, and affective. Working through the Study Guide, students will reinforce information presented in the textbook.

Special Features of the Study Guide

- **Chapter Objectives** focus on the major topics of the individual chapter information. Each objective addresses knowledge necessary for the entry-level medical assistant.

- **CAAHEP & ABHES Competencies** relevant to the chapter are listed at the start of the chapter.

- **Objective-Style Questions** include matching terms and definitions, defining major medical abbreviations, and multiple-choice format. Terminology and abbreviation review activities are a way for the student to review the major terms and abbreviations they may encounter during externship and into their employment in a medical facility.

- **Brief Answer Questions and Case Study Responses** require students to review the textbook chapter for essential information to the brief answer questions. The case study responses allow students to apply problem solving to case studies based on actual scenarios that may occur in the medical facility.

- **Internet Research** exercises encourage students to find more information about topics and subjects included in each chapter. Students learn how to access reliable Web sites to obtain additional information that will help them understand medical conditions and develop patient education materials.

- **Procedures Skill Sheets** provide students with the step-by-step process for performing the basic clinical skills they may encounter in the medical facility. Instructors can evaluate students assigning points for each step performed correctly. Students also are able to determine the amount of time to complete each procedure from start to finish. This finding teaches the student time management for their future work as a medical assistant.

The Study Guide has been developed to help students with their study and recall of information. Repetition has proven beneficial to the retention of information. Students can repeat the exercises to assist in remembering critical facts. It is also a great way to review prior to program examinations and ultimately the national certification examination. This *Study Guide for The Complete Medical Assistant* is an interactive tool ensuring students will access the textbook for review and to research the answers to the various exercises. The authors believe students will be challenged as they work their way through the Study Guide.

Contents

Section I

GENERAL SKILLS FOR THE MEDICAL ASSISTANT

1   Communication Skills for Medical Assistants   3

2   Law and Ethics   17

3   Medical Office Procedures   27

Section II

ANATOMY AND PHYSIOLOGY

4   Organization of the Body and Integumentary System   41

5   Skeletal and Muscular Systems   51

6   Nervous System, Special Senses, and Endocrine System   61

7   Digestive System and Nutrition   73

8   Cardiovascular and Respiratory Systems   83

9   Urinary and Reproductive Systems   93

Section III

ADMINISTRATIVE MEDICAL ASSISTANT SKILLS

10   Appointments and Schedules   105

11   Medical Documentation   117

12   Medical Insurance Coding   127

13   Managing Medical Office Finances   139

14   Health Insurance and Processing Claims   155

Section IV

CLINICAL MEDICAL ASSISTANT SKILLS

15   Medical Asepsis and Infection Control   169

16   Medical History and Patient Assessment   185

17   Assisting with the Physical Examination   209

18   Assisting with Minor Office Surgery   235

19   Pharmacology and Drug Administration   275

20   Diagnostic Testing   303

21   Patient Education   319

22   Medical Office Emergencies and Emergency Preparedness   331

Section V   ## CLINICAL LABORATORY

23   Medical Assistant Role in the Clinical Laboratory   347

24   Hematology   359

25   Phlebotomy   375

26   Immunology and Immunohematology   391

27   Urinalysis   405

28   Clinical Chemistry   423

29   Microbiology   437

Section I

General Skills for the Medical Assistant

1 Communication Skills for Medical Assistants

Chapter Objectives

- Recognize and respond to verbal communications.
- Identify and describe six interviewing skills.
- Recognize and respond to nonverbal communications.
- Describe the skill of active listening.
- List special techniques to use when talking to children and patients who are impaired or emotionally upset.
- Summarize how to act professionally in your communications with patients and with other health care providers.
- Identify community resources.
- Explain why having a professional image in the office is important.
- List the duties of a medical office receptionist.
- Explain general office policies.
- Demonstrate telephone techniques.
- Identify the common types of incoming calls and explain how to handle each type.
- Describe how to triage incoming calls.
- Explain how to identify and handle calls that involve medical emergencies.
- Respond to and initiate written communications.
- List six key guidelines for medical writing.
- Summarize how to write a business letter.
- Name the ways written materials can be sent and explain how each method is used.
- Describe the process for handling incoming mail.
- Demonstrate proper patient education technique.
- Summarize the theories of Maslow, Erikson, and Kubler-Ross.

CAAHEP & ABHES Competencies

CAAHEP

- Identify styles and types of verbal communication.
- Identify types of nonverbal communication.
- Recognize barriers to communication.
- Identify techniques for overcoming communication barriers.
- Recognize the elements of oral communication using a sender–receiver process.
- Define coaching a patient as it relates to health maintenance, disease prevention, compliance with treatment plan, community resources, and adaptations relevant to individual patient needs.
- Recognize elements of fundamental writing skills.
- Discuss applications of electronic technology in professional communication.
- Define the principles of self-boundaries.
- Define patient navigator.
- Describe the role of the medical assistant as a patient navigator.
- Relate the following behaviors to professional communication: assertive, aggressive, and passive.
- Differentiate between adaptive and nonadaptive coping mechanisms.
- Differentiate between subjective and objective information.
- Discuss the theories of Maslow, Erikson, and Kubler-Ross.
- Discuss examples of diversity (cultural, social, and ethnic).
- Use feedback techniques to obtain patient information.
- Respond to nonverbal communication.
- Use medical terminology correctly and pronounced accurately to communicate information to providers and patients.
- Coach patients regarding office policies, health maintenance, disease prevention, and treatment plans.
- Explain cultural diversity, developmental life stage, and communication barriers.
- Demonstrate professional telephone techniques.
- Document telephone messages accurately.
- Respond to nonverbal communication.
- Compose professional correspondence utilizing electronic technology.
- Develop a current list of community resources related to patients' health care needs.
- Facilitate referrals to community resources in the role of a patient navigator.
- Report relevant information concisely and accurately.

ABHES

- Display professionalism through written and verbal communications.
- Effectively screen patients' needs by utilizing effective communication.
- Assist in accurate patient education.
- Demonstrate the ability to teach patients self-examination, disease management, and health promotion.
- Perform the essential requirements for employment such as resume writing, effective interviewing, dressing professionally, time management, and following up appropriately.
- Demonstrate professional behavior.

TERMINOLOGY MATCHING

Directions: Match the terms in Column A with the definitions in Column B.

Column A

1. _____ Adaptive mechanism
2. _____ Aggressive
3. _____ Assertive
4. _____ Bias

5. _____ Clarification

6. _____ Communication
7. _____ Discrimination
8. _____ Established patient
9. _____ Feedback
10. _____ Grief

11. _____ Kinesics

12. _____ New patient
13. _____ Nonadaptive mechanism
14. _____ Objective

15. _____ Patient navigator
16. _____ Prejudice
17. _____ Proxemics

18. _____ Referral
19. _____ Stat
20. _____ Stereotyping

Column B

a. Represents a form of stereotyping
b. Used to ensure understanding of a message
c. The ability to learn to adjust to changes and thrive
d. Someone who has never been seen by the physician or other licensed provider within the practice or a patient who has not been seen or treated by the physician or other licensed provider within the practice in over 3 years
e. Holding an opinion about all members of a group based on oversimplified views about some of its members
f. Personal opinions about something
g. The study of body movements
h. Confident and forceful
i. Sending a response to a message expressing understanding
j. To treat people differently because of their backgrounds, cultures, or personal values
k. Person responsible for guiding the patient through the health care system
l. Inability to cope with changes such as increased stress
m. Refers to a person's "comfort zone"
n. A patient who has seen the physician before (within the last 3 years)
o. The sending and receiving of information
p. Immediately
q. When physician sends a patient to another office for special treatments, tests, or services
r. Great sadness
s. Information gained by observation or examination
t. Hostile or pushy

DEFINING ABBREVIATIONS

Directions: Provide the specific meaning of each of the following abbreviations. Watch your spelling.

21. ADA: _____

_____

22. FH: _____

_____

23. HIPAA: _____

_____

24. PMH: _____

_____

25. SH: _____

_____

MAKING IT RIGHT

Each of the following statements is false. Rewrite the statement to make it a true statement.

26. Clarifying is making sure you answer patients' questions and concerns.

_____

_____

_____

_____

27. The best guidelines for professional communication include speaking in a professional manner, using slang expressions, and talking down to patients.

_____

_____

_____

_____

28. Sighs, sobs, and laughs are examples of paralanguage.

_____

_____

_____

_____

29. Adapting is stating your message in a clear and direct way.

_____

_____

_____

_____

30. Kinesics refers to a person's comfort zone.

_____

_____

_____

_____

MULTIPLE CHOICE

Directions: Choose the best answer for each question.

31. The study of body movements is:

    a. proxemics.
    b. kinesics.
    c. adapting.
    d. passive.
    e. bias.

32. An individual's core values and beliefs are shaped by their:

    a. environment.
    b. bias.
    c. education level.
    d. income level.
    e. culture.

33. The ability to adjust to changes and thrive even in the most stressful situation is referred to as:

    a. adaptive mechanisms.
    b. adaptive processes.
    c. nonadaptive mechanisms.
    d. nonadaptive processes.
    e. adaptive measures.

34. When a physician sends a patient to another office for specialist services or testing, this action is called a:

    a. ordering.
    b. referencing.
    c. referral.
    d. renewal.
    e. preauthorizing.

35. The art of dealing with people in difficult situations without offending them is termed:

    a. courtesy.
    b. manners.
    c. ethics.
    d. diplomacy.
    e. respect.

36. As a medical assistant, your patients will depend on you to guide them through the health care system. This role is referred to as a:

    a. patient navigator.
    b. patient advocate.
    c. role model.
    d. home care assistant.
    e. nursing assistant.

37. In communication, your posture or facial expressions send important messages beyond the spoken word and are referred to as:

    a. verbal communication.
    b. nonverbal communication.
    c. paralanguage.
    d. nonlanguage sounds.
    e. sign language.

38. The tone, volume, and pitch of voice are referred to as:

    a. verbal communication.
    b. nonverbal communication.
    c. paralanguage.
    d. nonlanguage sounds.
    e. sign language.

39. Facial expressions, gestures, and eye movement are studied in:

    a. proxemics.
    b. sign language.
    c. nonlanguage sounds.
    d. paralanguage.
    e. kinesics.

40. In communication, _____ is stating your message in a clear and direct way.

    a. validating
    b. adapting
    c. clarifying
    d. reasoning
    e. questioning

41. _____ is insuring that your message answers the patient's questions or concerns.

    a. validating
    b. adapting
    c. clarifying
    d. questioning
    e. reasoning

42. What is the process of keeping the patient's level of understanding in mind when communicating?

    a. Validating
    b. Adapting
    c. Clarifying
    d. Questioning
    e. Reasoning

43. Which of the skills below is used in this communication: "We will contact you with the results of your Pap smear. Do you have any further questions I can answer?"

    a. Validating
    b. Adapting
    c. Clarifying
    d. Questioning
    e. Reasoning

44. Which of the following terms refers to how a person reacts to others in the space around them, or one's "personal space"?

    a. Kinesics
    b. Paralanguage
    c. Nonadaptive behavior
    d. Adaptive behavior
    e. Proxemics

45. What questions should you address when composing an informative letter?

    a. How, who, can, where, and did
    b. Who, what, where, when, and why
    c. Possibly, could, would, how, and when
    d. What, can, will, why, and possibly
    e. Where, would, how, who, and why

46. What are the three basic ways to organize information in a letter?

    a. Chronological
    b. Problem oriented
    c. Comparison
    d. All of the above
    e. Chronological, financial, and detailed

47. The process of checking spelling, grammar, punctuation, and accuracy of information in a letter is called:

    a. composing.
    b. planning.
    c. editing.
    d. preparing.
    e. organizing.

48. Memorandums differ from letter in that they:

    a. have a dateline.
    b. don't use salutations or closing.
    c. have a subject or reference line.
    d. don't have a dateline.
    e. don't use a subject or reference line.

49. What part of a letter is placed two to four lines below the letterhead?

    a. Inside address
    b. Subject line
    c. Salutation
    d. Body
    e. Date

50. This optional part of a letter is placed on the third line below the inside address, if used.

    a. Subject line
    b. Letterhead
    c. Inside address
    d. Date
    e. Salutation

51. When the letter "c" appears at the bottom of a letter, it indicates:

    a. the purpose of the letter is collections.
    b. a copy of the letter has been sent somewhere else.
    c. the purpose of the letter is to dispute charges.
    d. a copy of the letter will be retained on file.
    e. the letter was composed on a computer.

52. The part of a letter that contains the name, address, and phone and fax numbers of the physician's office or practice is referred to as the:

    a. subject line.
    b. salutation.
    c. letterhead.
    d. date.
    e. inside address.

53. The name and address of the individual receiving the letter is referred to as the:

    a. subject line.
    b. salutation.
    c. letterhead.
    d. date.
    e. inside address.

54. The salutation of a letter should be placed:

    a. two spaces below the inside address or subject line.
    b. four spaces below the inside address or date.
    c. four spaces below the letterhead or subject line.
    d. two spaces below the date or letterhead.
    e. four spaces below the inside address or subject line.

55. Where is the closing of the letter placed?

    a. Two spaces below the inside address.
    b. Two spaces below the subject line.
    c. Two spaces below the body of the letter.
    d. Two spaces below the letterhead.
    e. Two spaces below the date.

56. Which of the following rules apply to the body of the letter?

    a. It should be double spaced with triple spacing between paragraphs.
    b. Letter head should be used for all pages of the letter.
    c. Single spacing should be used with double spacing between paragraphs.
    d. Plain paper, not letterhead, should be used for all pages.
    e. None of the above are correct.

57. The abbreviation "Enc" at the end of letter indicates:

    a. something is included with the letter.
    b. special delivery of the letter.
    c. additional action in response to the letter is required.
    d. the contents of the envelope are confidential.
    e. a return signature is needed.

58. When sending information via fax, a cover sheet should also be used. The cover sheet should contain which of the following?

    a. Name, address, and phone and fax number of the office sending the fax
    b. Name of the person to receive the fax, fax number, and phone number
    c. Date and number of pages being sent
    d. Confidentiality statement
    e. All of the above

59. Which of the following are important steps to remember when creating your resume?

    a. It should appear in ascending order with the most recent events appearing first.
    b. Your resume should be flashy and artful regardless of the position you seek.
    c. Content is more important than accuracy of spelling or grammar.
    d. Embellish your resume with skills, education, and employment that aren't true to get your foot in the door.
    e. It should be multiple pages to show the employer how valuable you are.

60. A letter of application gives you the opportunity to:

    a. ask questions about pay.
    b. opens the door to communication about benefits.
    c. learn more about the position and the company.
    d. explain why you are interested in the position and what makes you the best candidate.
    e. discuss your hobbies and what you like to do when you're not working.

BRIEF EXPLANATIONS

61. Describe three ADA building requirements that must be met to ensure proper access to those with disabilities.

    _____

    _____

    _____

    _____

62. Patients with certain contagious diseases should not be left in waiting room where they would expose others. List four contagious diseases that would require moving the patient out of the waiting room and give a brief description as to how you would recognize each disease.

    _____

    _____

    _____

    _____

63. Upon arrival to the office, name four things the receptionist should do prior to the arrival of the first patient.

    _____

    _____

    _____

    _____

64. List five guidelines you should follow to maintain a professional appearance.

    _____

    _____

    _____

    _____

65. Describe three things you can do to show courtesy and respect to your coworkers.

_____

_____

_____

_____

66. Explain three ways that you, as a medical assistant, can influence a patient's view of the physician and office.

_____

_____

_____

_____

WHAT DO YOU DO?

67. Read the following scenario and respond to the questions with a short answer.

You've been searching for the perfect job. Your friend calls to tell you that the office he works in is now hiring. You really want to work at in this office because of all the wonderful things you have heard from employees and patients.

a. What course of action should you take first?

_____

_____

_____

_____

b. During the interview, the office manager asks why she should hire you over other candidates. What is your response?

_____

_____

_____

_____

c. During the interview, you are asked the following questions; please record your responses below. Have you or will you be taking a certification exam? What is, or will be, your credential? Where do you see yourself in 5 years? Why do you want to work here?

_____

_____

_____

_____

d. You are offered the position; however, the pay is much less than you thought it would be. They do offer excellent benefits that will save you some money. What should you do?

_____

_____

_____

_____

PATIENT EDUCATION

68. Write a short narrative script that you can use to provide EMS with important information regarding a patient that went into cardiac arrest at the office. Other team members are performing CPR with an AED while you contact EMS.

_____

_____

_____

_____

INTERNET RESEARCH

Visit the Mayo Clinic Web site at http://www.mayoclinic.org/patient-care-and-health-information, and research GERD. Identify specific signs, symptoms, and treatments available to patients. Create an outline that will help you in educating patients on GERD.

_____

_____

_____

_____

_____

_____

_____

Procedure 1-1 | Documenting Patient Education

Name: _____ Date: _____ Time: _____ Grade:_____

Equipment: Computer with an EHR program.

Performance Requirement: Student will perform this skill with ____% accuracy not to exceed _____ minutes. (Instructor will determine the point value for each step, % accuracy, and minutes required.)

Performance Checklist

Point Value	Performance Points Earned	Procedure Steps
		1. Obtain an electronic copy of printed materials that the patient will receive.
		2. In the patient's EHR, record the date, time, subject of education provided, and the names of those present during the education.
		3. Document, in detail, the manner information was presented.
		4. Evaluate the effectiveness of your teaching and record the results of the instruction.
		5. Document information regarding future appointments, evaluations, or follow-up reports.

CALCULATION

Total Points Possible: _____

Total Points Earned: _____

Points Earned/Points Possible = _____%

Student completion time (minutes): _____

PASS   FAIL   COMMENTS:

_____

Student's signature _____ Date _____

Instructor's signature _____ Date _____

Procedure 1-2 | Explaining General Office Procedures and Policies to the Patient

Name: _____ Date: _____ Time: _____ Grade: _____

Equipment: The General Office Procedure and Policies brochure, highlighter, business card, and pen.

Performance Requirement: Student will perform this skill with ____% accuracy not to exceed _____ minutes. (Instructor will determine the point value for each step, % accuracy, and minutes required.)

Performance Checklist

Point Value	Performance Points Earned	Procedure Steps
		1. Welcome the patient to the practice. Introduce yourself to the patient and explain your role in the office.
		2. Review the office brochure with the patient. Highlight areas of importance such as: office hours, appointment scheduling, prescription refills, and after hours contact.
		3. Answer any questions the patient may have. Encourage the patient to contact you if they have questions after they leave.
		4. Give the brochure to the patient along with a business card. Write your name and contact information on the back.
		5. Document the review of policies in the patient's record.

CALCULATION

Total Points Possible: _____

Total Points Earned: _____

Points Earned/Points Possible = _____%

Student completion time (minutes): _____

PASS   FAIL   COMMENTS:

_____

Student's signature _____ Date _____

Instructor's signature _____ Date _____

Procedure 1-3 | Writing a Professional Business Letter

Name: _____   Date: _____   Time: _____   Grade: _____

Equipment: Computer with word processing program, 8 ½ × 11 paper, a number 10 envelope, and the information below. Dr. Georgia Parks has asked you to compose a letter to patient, Dwayne Waterman, 12105 Quality Lane, Chesterfield, MO 63017, terminating the physician\patient relationship. She is terminating Mr. Waterman's care due to his noncompliance and failure to adhere to the narcotic use agreement he signed. Dr. Parks has advised you she will terminate the patient's care 15 days after the receipt of the letter. She will provide urgent and emergency care until that time. Dr. Parks also wants the patient informed that she will no longer prescribe any narcotic pain medications. She will release his medical records to the physician taking over his care upon receipt of a signed release of medical information. This letter will be sent certified with return receipt. Use block format, all line with start flush with the left margin.

Performance Requirement: Student will perform this skill with ____% accuracy not to exceed _____ minutes. (Instructor will determine the point value for each step, % accuracy, and minutes required.)

Performance Checklist

Point Value	Performance Points Earned	Procedure Steps
		1. Compose a rough draft of the body of the letter. Take time to ensure all the information needed is covered. Have others review the letter for content and accuracy. Be certain to follow proper format and spacing guidelines.
		2. Create a "header" to serve as letterhead for Dr. Georgia Parks and include a mailing address and phone number.
		3. Insert the date or dateline of your letter.
		4. Enter the inside address.
		5. Enter the subject line.
		6. Type the body of your letter.
		7. Select and enter your professional complimentary close.
		8. Enter the typed signature.
		9. Record the reference initials.

CALCULATION

Total Points Possible: _____

Total Points Earned: _____

Points Earned/Points Possible = _____%

Student completion time (minutes): _____

PASS   FAIL   COMMENTS:

_____

Student's signature _____   Date _____

Instructor's signature _____   Date _____

2 Law and Ethics

Chapter Objectives

- Explain why knowledge of law and ethics is important when working in a medical facility.
- Describe the difference between law, ethics, etiquette, morals, and values.
- Distinguish how law and ethics are related.
- Compare the consequences of unlawful and unethical behavior.
- Define the three main sources of law.
- Describe the three different types of law.
- Compare and contrast criminal and civil law.
- Define *respondeat superior* and explain how it relates in a health care setting.
- Identify the three parts of a valid contract.
- Differentiate between expressed and implied contracts.
- List the steps a physician must follow when terminating a contract.
- Describe the medical assistant's scope of practice and explain resources available to answer medical assistant questions.
- Explain standard of care as it relates to physicians and medical assistants.
- Explain the difference between intentional and unintentional torts.
- Define and explain the difference between malfeasance, misfeasance, and nonfeasance.
- Identify the four Ds of negligence.

CAAHEP & ABHES Competencies

CAAHEP

- Identify and respond to issues of confidentiality.
- Perform within legal and ethical boundaries.
- Demonstrate knowledge of federal and state health care legislation and regulations.

ABHES

- Comply with federal, state, and local health laws and regulations as they relate to health care settings.
- Define scope of practice for the medical assistant within the state that the medical assistant is employed.

- Describe what procedures can and cannot be delegated to the medical assistant and by whom within various employment settings.
- Perform risk management procedures.
- Understand the importance of maintaining liability coverage once employed in the industry.
- Display compliance with code of ethics of the profession.
- Follow established policy in initiating or terminating medical treatment.

TERMINOLOGY MATCHING

Directions: Match the terms in Column A with the definitions in Column B.

Column A

1. _____ Abandonment
2. _____ Arbitration
3. _____ Assault
4. _____ Battery
5. _____ Beneficence
6. _____ Breach
7. _____ Contract
8. _____ Defendant
9. _____ Dilemma
10. _____ Embezzlement
11. _____ Ethics
12. _____ Etiquette
13. _____ Felonies
14. _____ Fidelity
15. _____ Fraud
16. _____ Integrity
17. _____ Libel
18. _____ Malfeasance
19. _____ Malpractice
20. _____ Misdemeanor
21. _____ Misfeasance
22. _____ Negligence
23. _____ Nonfeasance
24. _____ Plaintiff
25. _____ Precedents
26. _____ *Res ipsa loquitur*
27. _____ *Respondeat superior*
28. _____ Slander
29. _____ *Stare decisis*

Column B

a. Taking an improper action
b. Less serious crimes that are punishable by fines or short jail sentences
c. Threatening a person or acting in a way that causes the person to fear harm
d. Results from failing to act with reasonable care, causing harm to another person
e. Not taking a necessary action
f. Means doing good
g. Let the decision stand
h. Faithfulness and loyalty to others
i. A voluntary agreement between two parties from which each party benefits
j. Earlier decisions made in court cases
k. A problem caused by a conflict between choices
l. When a professional person is negligent in his or her duties
m. An alternative method to settle a dispute without going to court
n. Serious crimes that are punishable by long prison sentences or even by death
o. Order issued by the court to obtain evidence
p. Guidelines for determining proper behavior
q. Unlawful touching
r. Damaging a person's reputation in writing
s. Person accused of breaking the law
t. A failure to do what's required or what you have been expected to do under contract
u. The party that charges the wrongdoing
v. Taking a proper action but in an improper way
w. Speaking lies about another person that harms the person's reputation or employment
x. Occurs when the physician ends the relationship without proper notice while the patient still needs treatment
y. Any deceitful act with the intention of concealing the truth
z. The thing speaks for itself
aa. Wrongful taking of money or property that you're responsible for and using it for your own personal needs
bb. Laws passed by congress or by state legislatures
cc. A common law principle that employers are responsible for the actions of their employees

30. _____ Statutes
31. _____ Subpoena
32. _____ Tort

33. _____ Tortfeasor
34. _____ Veracity
35. _____ Verdict

dd. The person who commits the tort
ee. Rules for polite behavior
ff. Being truthful and honest
gg. Wrongs committed against a person or property that don't involve violation of a contract
hh. The quality of strongly sticking to your principles
ii. The decision of whether the defendant is guilty or innocent

DEFINING ABBREVIATIONS

Directions: Provide the specific meaning of each of the following abbreviations. Watch your spelling.

36. AAMA: _____

37. ABHES: _____

38. ADAAA: _____

39. AMT: _____

40. CAAHEP: _____

41. CMA: _____

42. DEA: _____

43. HHS: _____

44. HIPAA: _____

45. PHI: _____

46. PSDA: _____

47. RMA: _____

MAKING IT RIGHT

Each of the following statements is false. Rewrite the statement to make it a true statement.

48. Decisions from past cases are used as a guide to apply law to current cases. The legal principle for this is called *res ipsa loquitur* meaning "let the decision stand."

_____

_____

_____

_____

49. Each branch of government produces a different kind of law.
    - Statutory law comes from the executive branch.
    - The judicial branch creates administrative law.
    - Case law results from the actions of the legislative branch.

_____

_____

_____

_____

50. The physician is legally responsible for the actions of his/her medical assistant. Therefore, any errors made by a medical assistant would put the physician at risk. This legal principle is referred to as "*stare decisis*," which translates to "let the master answer."

_____

_____

_____

_____

MULTIPLE CHOICE

Directions: Choose the best answer for each question.

51. Which of the following regulates how your office handles and prescribes certain drugs?

    a. Controlled Substances Act
    b. Health Insurance Portability and Accountability Act
    c. False Claims Act
    d. Anti-Kickback Statute
    e. Stark Law

52. What government agency creates the regulatory processes to be followed under HIPAA?

    a. DEA
    b. ADAAA
    c. AMA
    d. AOA
    e. HHS

53. When a judge uses previous cases tried under the same law to determine how the law was applied it is called _____.

    a. *respondeat superior*
    b. *stare decisis*
    c. *res ipsa loquitur*
    d. *proximate cause*
    e. *dereliction of duty*

54. In a case where the mistake is so obvious that no more evidence is needed, such as a surgeon removing the noninfected leg on a patient, it is referred to as:

    a. *respondeat superior.*
    b. *stare decisis.*
    c. *res ipsa loquitur.*
    d. *proximate cause.*
    e. *dereliction of duty.*

55. When you explain to a patient that the physician has ordered labs that require drawing blood and the patient extends the arm out to you, this act is considered:

    a. expressed consent.
    b. implied consent.
    c. informed consent.
    d. written consent.
    e. procedural consent.

56. If a patient fails to follow the physician's orders and is in breach of contract, the physician may choose to end the patient–physician relationship. If the patient is not properly informed of this action in writing, the physician could be charged with:

    a. malfeasance.
    b. proximate cause.
    c. misfeasance.
    d. abandonment.
    e. direct cause.

57. A court order requiring medical records be presented to court would be referred to as a/an:

    a. subpoena duces tecum.
    b. summons.
    c. order.
    d. case law.
    e. administrative law.

58. When a person does good, especially doing things that will benefit others, it is called:

    a. ethics.
    b. humility.
    c. values.
    d. responsibility.
    e. beneficence.

59. The expression "put yourself in the person shoes" applies to which of the following?

    a. Sympathy
    b. Fidelity
    c. Empathy
    d. Veracity
    e. Integrity

60. Faithfulness and loyalty to others is:

    a. sympathy.
    b. fidelity.
    c. empathy.
    d. veracity.
    e. integrity.

61. _____ means to be truthful and honest.

    a. Sympathy
    b. Fidelity
    c. Empathy
    d. Veracity
    e. Integrity

62. The quality of strongly sticking to your principles is:

    a. sympathy.
    b. fidelity.
    c. empathy.
    d. veracity.
    e. integrity.

63. Which of the following means "fairness in actions toward all people"?

    a. Integrity
    b. Justice
    c. Tolerance
    d. Perseverance
    e. Honesty

64. _____ is showing respect for others opinions, beliefs, practices, or backgrounds even if they are different from your own.

    a. Tolerance
    b. Integrity
    c. Honesty
    d. Perseverance
    e. Justice

65. Which of the following terms means "being truthful in every situation"?

    a. Tolerance
    b. Justice
    c. Honesty
    d. Integrity
    e. Perseverance

66. Continuing with an action despite obstacles is _____.

    a. Tolerance
    b. Integrity
    c. Honesty
    d. Perseverance
    e. Justice

67. A _____ is the range of activities that a health care worker is qualified to perform.

    a. Job title
    b. Scope of practice
    c. License
    d. Certification
    e. Standard

68. Which of the following represents a common administrative task a medical assistant would perform?

    a. Obtaining patient medical histories
    b. Assisting the physician during examinations
    c. Performing waived laboratory tests
    d. Collecting and preparing laboratory specimens
    e. Handling correspondence, billing, and bookkeeping

69. Which of the following would represent a common clinical task a medical assistant would perform?

    a. Setting up referral appointments
    b. Answering phones and scheduling appointments
    c. Explaining treatment procedures to patients
    d. Arranging for hospital admissions and lab services
    e. Completing and submitting insurance claim forms

70. Which of the following represents the four "Ds" of negligence?

    a. Duty, dereliction of duty, direct cause, damages
    b. Duty, divergence, direct cause, damages
    c. Dereliction of duty, divergence, direct cause, damages
    d. Direct cause, deceit, duty, damages
    e. Damages, deceit, demeaning, dereliction of duty

BRIEF EXPLANATIONS

71. Describe the three branches of American government and their role in the making of laws.

    _____
    _____
    _____
    _____

72. Explain the difference between criminal law and civil law.

_____

_____

_____

_____

73. Provide examples of situations that would demonstrate each of the following:
slander, libel, assault, and battery.

_____

_____

_____

_____

WHAT DO YOU DO?

74. Read the following scenario and respond to the questions with a short answer.

Your office has recently hired a new billing and coding person, Julianne. She is nice and gets along well with everyone including the patients. One day, you hear Julianne explaining to a patient that a procedure that they are to have done is not covered by their insurance. The patient is very upset as she really wants this procedure. You hear Julianne tell the patient not to worry about because she will just change the procedure to something that is covered so the physician gets paid and the patient can have her procedure without paying 100% out of pocket.

a. What steps should you take to ensure that proper protocol is followed?

_____

_____

_____

_____

b. If you ignore this situation and the patient has the procedure with Julianne intentionally changing the codes to something, what can the physician be charge with?

_____

_____

_____

_____

c. If Julianne moves forward with her plan what can happen to her? If you elect to do nothing, what charges or actions could you be face with in the future?

_____

_____

_____

_____

d. You report the situation to the office manager and she seems excited to have someone that is willing to help patients get what they want, despite the fact that it is fraud. What would you do next?

_____

_____

_____

_____

PATIENT EDUCATION

75. Write a short narrative explaining the importance of obtaining patient consent prior to performing any procedure, including venipuncture. What tort could you be charged with if you perform a procedure despite the patient objecting?

_____

_____

_____

_____

INTERNET RESEARCH

Visit the IRS Web site https://www.irs.gov/uac/examples-of-healthcare-fraud-investigations-fiscal-year-2015 and research physicians or facilities charged with health care fraud. Select a case and compose a summary of the fraud and the actions taken against the individual(s).

_____

_____

_____

_____

_____

_____

_____

3 | Medical Office Procedures

Chapter Objectives

- Review functions of computers in the medical office.
- Explain the proper use and function of an organization's intranet.
- Discuss general guidelines for computerized appointment scheduling.
- Review various computer programs used within the health care environment.
- Discuss the importance of proper computer ethics.
- Create professional e-mails.
- Review guidelines for opening of e-mail attachments and potential hazards.
- Maintain password and computer security.
- Understand basic Internet safety and usage.
- Discuss the role and goals of quality improvement.
- Summarize the guidelines for completing incident reports.
- Perform an inventory of supplies and equipment.

CAAHEP & ABHES Competencies

CAAHEP

- Perform routine maintenance of administrative and clinical equipment.
- Perform an inventory with documentation.
- Explain the purpose of routine maintenance of administrative and clinical equipment.
- List steps involved in completing an inventory.
- Explain the importance of data backup.

ABHES

- Maintain inventory of equipment and supplies.
- Perform routine maintenance of administrative equipment.

TERMINOLOGY MATCHING

Directions: Match the terms in Column A with the definitions in Column B.

Column A

1. _____ Cookies
2. _____ Firewalls
3. _____ Incident reports
4. _____ Intranet
5. _____ Inventory
6. _____ Privileged information
7. _____ Risk management
8. _____ Service contract
9. _____ Unsecure information
10. _____ Viruses

Column B

a. Written accounts of negative events experienced by patients, visitors, or staff
b. Listing of the amounts and types of supplies/equipment on hand
c. Process of identifying and correcting problems before they cause injury
d. Information entered on a site that could potentially be viewed by others
e. Tiny files sites leave on a hard drive that track your online activity
f. All information pertaining to the medical care of a patient
g. Internal business system that provides quick access to company information
h. Can invade a computer system and destroy files and software
i. An arrangement with a company to care for office equipment for an agreed upon amount
j. Programs or devices that prevent unauthorized users from accessing the system

DEFINING ABBREVIATIONS

Directions: Provide the specific meaning of each of the following abbreviations. Watch your spelling.

11. CLIA: _____

_____

12. CMS: _____

_____

13. EHR/EMR: _____

_____

14. HHS: _____

_____

15. HIPAA: _____

_____

16. POL: _____

_____

17. QI: _____

_____

18. SSL: _____

_____

MAKING IT RIGHT

Each of the following statements is false. Rewrite the statement to make it a true statement.

19. Passwords are designed to be shared as there are a limited number available to the facility.

_____

_____

_____

_____

20. The **intranet** gives you access to the World Wide Web making it easy to access information for patient care.

_____

_____

_____

_____

21. The best way to notify the physician of an emergency is via e-mail.

_____

_____

_____

_____

22. When providing personal information over the Internet, it is important to ensure the site does not have an SSL.

_____

_____

_____

_____

23. HIPAA was created to monitor CLIA, CMS, and HHS.

_____

_____

_____

_____

MULTIPLE CHOICE

Directions: Choose the best answer for each question.

24. QI programs benefit health care organizations by:
    a. providing funds for underinsured patients.
    b. improving service to patients and their families.
    c. preventing unauthorized users from accessing your computer.
    d. allowing medical records to be faxed.
    e. tracking the current accounts receivable for your office.

25. The policy and procedure manuals for your facility could be quickly accessed using which of the following?

    a. Internet
    b. POL
    c. CLIA
    d. Intranet
    e. Secure sockets layer

26. Which of the following types of programs would you use to compose a letter to a patient?

    a. Word processing
    b. Accounting
    c. Scheduling
    d. Patient tracking
    e. Insurance submission

27. The standard to be followed for the security and privacy of patients' health care information is:

    a. CLIA.
    b. HIPAA.
    c. CMAS.
    d. POL.
    e. OSHA.

28. What are the three levels of complexity under CLIA?

    a. Waived, standard, and high
    b. Low, medium, and high
    c. Waived, moderate, and restricted
    d. Low, moderate, and restricted
    e. Waived, moderate, and high

29. Which of the following grants approval for clinical laboratory testing?

    a. CMS
    b. HHS
    c. OSHA
    d. CLIA
    e. POL

30. Performing a urine dipstick would fall under which of the following CLIA complexities?

    a. Moderate
    b. Restricted
    c. High
    d. Low
    e. Waived

31. Performing a packaged rapid strep test would fall under which of the following CLIA complexities?

    a. Moderate
    b. Restricted
    c. High
    d. Low
    e. Waived

32. Performance of a Gram stain would fall under which CLIA complexity?

    a. Moderate
    b. Restricted
    c. High
    d. Low
    e. Waived

33. Under which CLIA complexity would you find centrifuged microhematocrits?

    a. Moderate
    b. Restricted
    c. High
    d. Low
    e. Waived

34. Urine pregnancy testing would be which of the following complexities?

    a. Moderate
    b. Restricted
    c. High
    d. Low
    e. Waived

35. When viewing information online, some sites leave tiny files on your hard
    drive that track your activity; these tiny files are referred to as:

    a. firewalls.
    b. cookies.
    c. viruses.
    d. secure sockets layer.
    e. unsecure information.

36. An incident report would be completed in which of the following situations?

    a. A patient presents with a swollen ankle after falling down the stairs in her apartment building.
    b. The guest of a patient complains that the coffee in the waiting room is too strong.
    c. A patient receives the wrong injection and has an allergic reaction.
    d. The physician is angry because the wrong supplies were ordered.
    e. An employee arrives 30 minutes early to work to get a head start on a busy day.

37. Your office purchased an agreement with a company to come every 6 months
    to do preventative maintenance and repairs on the laboratory equipment. This
    agreement is referred to as a:

    a. purchase order.
    b. purchase agreement.
    c. service contract.
    d. service order.
    e. requisition order.

38. When creating a password, which of the following would be appropriate?

    a. Tape the password to your computer so you have it in case your forget it.
    b. Use your name and birth date so it will easily be remembered.
    c. Use a combination of capital and lower case letters along with numbers.
    d. Make things simple and use "password."
    e. Avoid changing your password.

39. When performing a supply inventory, which of the following should be noted?

    a. Expiration dates
    b. Brand names and serial numbers
    c. Quantity
    d. All of the above
    e. Delivery fees

40. Which of the following would be an example of a POL?

    a. Hospital laboratory
    b. Medical office laboratory
    c. Reference laboratory
    d. Independent laboratory
    e. State laboratory

41. Which of the following maintain the standards of care in both the clinical and administrative areas of health care?

    a. OSHA and CLIA
    b. CMS and HIPAA
    c. OSHA and POL
    d. CLIA and HIPAA
    e. POL and CMS

42. Prior to sharing any information online you should look for what symbol to indicate that it is a secure site?

    a. Open lock
    b. Closed lock
    c. Key
    d. Cloud
    e. Question mark

43. A firewall helps protect against viruses by:

    a. allowing access to all Internet sites.
    b. limiting access to specific Internet sites.
    c. allowing access to any files on a site.
    d. limiting the amount of time spent on a site.
    e. performing scans on every site prior to opening it.

44. Which of the following sets standards for submitting claims to patients' health insurers?

    a. HIPPA
    b. OSHA
    c. CLIA
    d. POL
    e. HIPAA

45. Why did congress pass CLIA in 1988?

    a. To generate additional funds for the laboratories
    b. To generate additional government funds
    c. Because results were inaccurate and people were dying
    d. Because congress wanted to control the labs
    e. To promote the work of laboratories

46. What is the title of the person who is responsible for insuring HIPAA requirements are followed in the office?

    a. Insurance manager
    b. Privacy officer
    c. Information specialist
    d. Insurance officer
    e. Privacy specialist

47. Which of the following would be a risk factor?

    a. Secure mats in the entry
    b. Well-lit parking lot and entry
    c. Frayed electrical wires on an ECG machine
    d. The use of secured sharps containers
    e. Requiring photo identification of patients

48. Most insurance companies have Web sites that medical facilities can use to access information. Which of the following would you be able to access from such a site?

    a. Patient eligibility
    b. Individual policy benefits
    c. Preauthorization of a medication or service
    d. Status of submitted claims
    e. All of the above

BRIEF EXPLANATIONS

49. List precautions you can take to help prevent viruses on your computer system.

    _____

    _____

    _____

    _____

50. Explain why CLIA was necessary and what affect it has had on health care.

    _____

    _____

    _____

    _____

51. List three procedures that can be performed under waived testing.

    _____

    _____

    _____

    _____

52. List three procedures that can be performed under CLIA's moderate complexity.

_____

_____

_____

_____

53. List four ways the QI can benefit health care organizations.

_____

_____

_____

_____

54. Computer systems are vital to the day-to-day functions in the medical office. List three functions that are essential for daily operations.

_____

_____

_____

_____

55. List four pieces of information that you should check when completing an inventory or supply order.

_____

_____

_____

_____

WHAT DO YOU DO?

56. Read the following scenario and respond to the questions with a short answer.

Your office has strict rules regarding the moving of office equipment, including computers. You love the sun; however, your desk is across the room from direct sun expose. You measure and discover you have more than enough cord and wires to reach. So, you moved your desk and computer so that you could be in direct sunlight. A month or so after the move, your computer begins to overheat and shuts down at least twice a day. This never happened before.

a. What is your immediate thought as to the cause of this issue? What do you do first?

_____

_____

_____

_____

b. How do you explain this issue to your supervisor?

_____

_____

_____

_____

c. What issues could you face as a result of this action?

_____

_____

_____

_____

d. As a result of this needle puncture, what does your employer need to do?

_____

_____

_____

_____

57. The computer system in the office goes offline. You are unable to access vital information needed for the proper flow of the office. It's the middle of the day and you have a completely booked schedule. Your waiting room is full as our patient care rooms.

a. What is your first priority? How will this help the situation?

_____

_____

_____

_____

b. What steps can you take to ensure that patient care continues? How will you ensure the best possible care?

_____

_____

_____

_____

c. Describe how you inform patients of the situation while maintaining their trust in the care they will receive.

_____

_____

_____

_____

PATIENT EDUCATION

58. Write a short narrative script that you can use to walk a patient through the progress of obtaining and completing paperwork for prescription medication assistance from the drug manufacturer.

_____

_____

_____

_____

INTERNET RESEARCH

Visit the American Medical Association Web site at www.ama-assn.org and review guidelines and recommendations for successful participation in the Merit-based Incentive Program under the CMS MACRA (Medicare Access & CHIP Reauthorization Act). Describe actions you can implement to assist the physician with success compliance.

_____

_____

_____

_____

_____

_____

_____

_____

Procedure 3-1 | Conducting an Inventory of Supplies

Name: _____ Date: _____ Time: _____ Grade: _____

Equipment: Supply inventory sheets, requisition/order forms, and pen.

Performance Requirement: Student will perform this skill with _____% accuracy not to exceed _____ minutes. (Instructor will determine the point value for each step, % accuracy, and minutes required.)

Performance Checklist

Point Value	Performance Points Earned	Procedure Steps
		1. Create a list of supplies (administrative, clinical, and laboratory) used in your office.
		2. Determine par or minimum levels for each item on the supply list.
		3. Document current amounts on hand.
		4. Determine the amount needed by subtracting the par from the amount on hand.
		5. Complete the requisition/order form for supplies needed.
		6. Submit the requisition/order form to your office manager.
		7. Document actions taken.

CALCULATION

Total Points Possible: _____

Total Points Earned: _____

Points Earned/Points Possible = _____%

Student completion time (minutes): _____

PASS   FAIL   COMMENTS:

_____

Student's signature _____ Date _____

Instructor's signature _____ Date _____

Procedure 3-2 | Performing Routine Equipment Maintenance

Name: _____ Date: _____ Time: _____ Grade: _____

Equipment: Office equipment, lint-free towel, water, mild soap, other supplies as listed by manufacturer guidelines, and an equipment maintenance log.

Performance Requirement: Student will perform this skill with _____% accuracy not to exceed _____ minutes. (Instructor will determine the point value for each step, % accuracy, and minutes required.)

Performance Checklist

Point Value	Performance Points Earned	Procedure Steps
		1. Review manufacturer guidelines of your office equipment.
		2. Clean the exterior of the equipment.
		3. Perform maintenance step provided in the user's manual.
		4. Record maintenance completed for each piece of equipment on the maintenance log.
		5. Report any concerns discovered during these checks should be reported to your supervisor immediately.

CALCULATION

Total Points Possible: _____

Total Points Earned: _____

Points Earned/Points Possible = _____%

Student completion time (minutes): _____

PASS   FAIL   COMMENTS:

_____

Student's signature _____ Date _____

Instructor's signature _____ Date _____

Section II

Anatomy and Physiology

4 Organization of the Body and Integumentary System

Chapter Objectives

- Define the terms anatomy, physiology, and pathology.
- Describe the organization of the body from chemicals to the whole organism.
- List 11 body systems, and give the general function of each.
- Define and give examples of homeostasis.
- Using examples, discuss the components of a negative feedback loop.
- Define metabolism, and name the two types of metabolic reactions.
- List and define the main directional terms for the body.
- List and define the three planes of division of the body.
- Name the subdivisions of the dorsal and ventral cavities.
- Name and locate the subdivisions of the abdomen.
- Cite some anterior and posterior body regions along with their common names.
- Show how word parts are used to build words related to the body's organization.
- Name and describe the layers of the skin.
- Provide the location and function of the accessory structures of the integumentary system.
- List the major functions of the integumentary system.
- List the main disorders of the integumentary system.
- Describe the classification and danger of burns.

CAAHEP & ABHES Competencies

CAAHEP

- Describe structural organization of the human body.
- Identify body systems.
- Describe body planes, directional terms, quadrants, and body cavities.
- List major organs in each body system.
- Describe the normal function of each body system.

- Identify common pathology related to each body system including signs, symptoms, and etiology.
- Analyze pathology for each body system including diagnostic measures and treatment modalities.

ABHES

- List all body systems and their structure and functions.
- Describe common diseases, symptoms, and etiologies as they apply to each system.
- Common diseases, diagnoses, and treatments.
- Identify diagnostic and treatment modalities as they relate to each body system.

TERMINOLOGY MATCHING

Part I Directions: Match the terms in Column A with the definitions in Column B.

Column A

1. _____ Anabolism
2. _____ Anatomy
3. _____ Catabolism
4. _____ Extracellular fluid
5. _____ Homeostasis
6. _____ Intracellular fluid
7. _____ Metabolism
8. _____ Negative feedback
9. _____ Physiology

Column B

a. The sum of all chemical and physical changes that occur in the body's tissues
b. Fluid found outside the body's cells
c. The study of the function of the body parts
d. The breakdown of complex substances into simpler compounds
e. The steady state (sameness) within an organism
f. The study of the structure of the body
g. The building up of tissues through growth and repair
h. Fluid found inside of or within a cell
i. A method that reverses any shift from normal range by upward or downward changes

Part II Directions: Match the terms in Column A with the definitions in Column B.

Column A

10. _____ Adipose
11. _____ Albinism
12. _____ Cerumen
13. _____ Cyanosis
14. _____ Dermatosis
15. _____ Epidermis
16. _____ Erythema
17. _____ Impetigo
18. _____ Jaundice
19. _____ Keratin
20. _____ Melanin
21. _____ Melanoma
22. _____ Psoriasis
23. _____ Sebum
24. _____ Urticaria
25. _____ Vitiligo

Column B

a. Skin infection caused from a staphylococcal bacteria
b. Overgrowth of keratinocytes in the epidermis causing large areas of red flat areas that appear covered with silvery scales
c. Fatty tissue
d. Bluish discoloration when there is not enough oxygen in the blood
e. Hives caused from an allergic reaction
f. The top layer of the skin and contains no blood vessels
g. Hardened protein that forms fingernails and toenails
h. Malignant tumor of melanocytes
i. Destroys all forms of microorganisms, including bacterial spores
j. Lack of pigment in the skin, hair, and eyes
k. Ear wax
l. Yellowish skin discoloration, which may be caused by excessive amounts of bile pigments
m. Redness of the skin
n. General term used for any skin disease
o. Skin's main pigment produced by melanocytes
p. Oil that lubricates the skin and hair preventing dryness

DEFINING ABBREVIATIONS

Directions: Provide the specific meaning of each of the following abbreviations. Watch your spelling.

26. BSA: _____

_____

27. HPV: _____

_____

28. SLE: _____

_____

MAKING IT RIGHT

Each of the following statements is false. Rewrite the statement to make it a true statement.

29. Ligaments are the structures that attach muscle to bone and tendons join bone to bone.

_____

_____

_____

_____

30. Veins carry blood away from the heart and arteries carry blood to the heart.

_____

_____

_____

_____

31. The accessory organs of the digestive system include the appendix, esophagus, and pylorus.

_____

_____

_____

_____

32. Homeostasis is a term that means the body is in a constant state of change.

_____

_____

_____

_____

33. The term anterior means toward the lower part of the body and posterior means above the upper part of the body.

_____

_____

_____

_____

34. The epigastric region is centrally located just inferior to the umbilical region.

_____

_____

_____

35. Cyanosis refers to a yellowish skin discoloration and jaundice is a bluish discoloration of the skin.

_____

_____

_____

MULTIPLE CHOICE

Directions: Choose the best answer for each question.

36. A blister or fluid filled sac is a:

    a. macule.
    b. vesicle.
    c. nodule.
    d. pustule.
    e. ulcer.

37. A first-degree burn:

    a. is very painful due to nerve and tissue damage.
    b. penetrates the tissue to the subcutaneous layer.
    c. has watery blisters.
    d. appears reddened.
    e. requires skin grafting.

38. A mole is known as a:

    a. melanoma.
    b. nevus.
    c. fissure.
    d. papule.
    e. blemish.

39. The thoracic cavity and the abdominopelvic cavity are separated by the:

    a. mediastinum.
    b. pleura.
    c. diaphragm.
    d. stomach.
    e. peritoneum.

40. Which of these organs is located in the pelvic cavity?

    a. Stomach
    b. Liver
    c. Gallbladder
    d. Urinary bladder
    e. Pancreas

41. Which region is located inferior to the umbilical region?

    a. Hypogastric
    b. Epigastric
    c. Hypochondriac
    d. Lumbar
    e. Iliac

42. A type of infection caused from staphylococcal bacteria is:

    a. varicella.
    b. fissure.
    c. vesicle.
    d. herpes.
    e. impetigo.

43. Which of these is responsible for causing mycotic infections?

    a. Bacteria
    b. Virus
    c. Fungus
    d. Helminth
    e. Parasite

44. Wheals are present when the patient has:

    a. a bacterial infection.
    b. ringworm.
    c. shingles.
    d. allergies.
    e. acne.

45. Systemic lupus erythematosus is a chronic disease, which is:

    a. caused from an overgrowth of keratinocytes in the epidermis.
    b. an autoimmune disease of connective tissue.
    c. the result of oversecretion of sebum from sebaceous glands.
    d. a viral infection that causes watery blisters on the torso of the body.
    e. caused by a systemic fungal infection.

46. What fungal condition is encouraged to grow with dampness and perspiration?

    a. Athlete's foot
    b. Herpes zoster
    c. Impetigo
    d. Urticaria
    e. Psoriasis

47. Which directional terms are accurately paired together?

    a. Anterior and inferior
    b. Posterior and medial
    c. Superior and inferior
    d. Lateral and dorsal
    e. Ventral and proximal

48. A primary function of the urinary system is to:

    a. increase the body's metabolism.
    b. remove carbon dioxide from the blood.
    c. produce red blood cells.
    d. remove waste products from the blood.
    e. produce bile to metabolize fats.

49. Internal body temperature control is located in a region of the:

    a. brain.
    b. heart.
    c. skin.
    d. kidneys.
    e. liver.

50. The elbow is located:

    a. distal to the wrist.
    b. proximal to the shoulder.
    c. inferior to the hand.
    d. superior to the shoulder.
    e. proximal to the wrist.

51. The coronal plane is also known as the:

    a. sagittal plane.
    b. frontal plane.
    c. midsagittal plane.
    d. dorsal plane.
    e. transverse plane.

52. The hypochondriac regions are located:

    a. superior to the thoracic cavity.
    b. lateral to the inguinal regions.
    c. inferior to the ribs.
    d. medial to the lumbar regions.
    e. superior to the mediastinum.

53. A structure located in the right lower quadrant is the:

    a. appendix.
    b. spleen.
    c. liver.
    d. stomach.
    e. pancreas.

54. The three layers of the skin include the:

    a. dermis and adipose layers.
    b. subcutaneous and dermis layers.
    c. epidermis and endodermis layers.
    d. adipose and subcutaneous layers.
    e. epidermis and adipose layers.

55. The protein substance that thickens and protects the skin is:

    a. sebum.
    b. melanin.
    c. adipose.
    d. cellulite.
    e. keratin.

56. The fatty tissue that acts as insulation and provides a reserve energy supply is:

    a. sebum.
    b. melanin.
    c. adipose.
    d. cellulite.
    e. keratin.

57. Sudoriferous glands secrete:

    a. sebum.
    b. sweat.
    c. cerumen.
    d. melanin.
    e. keratin.

58. A rough, jagged wound caused by tearing the skin is:

    a. an ulcer.
    b. a vesicle.
    c. a laceration.
    d. a fissure.
    e. a macule.

59. Varicella is also known as:

    a. chickenpox.
    b. impetigo.
    c. papillomavirus.
    d. tinea corporis.
    e. urticaria.

60. A common disorder caused by oversecretion of oil from the sebaceous glands is:

   a. impetigo.
   b. psoriasis.
   c. eczema.
   d. athlete's foot.
   e. acne vulgaris.

BRIEF EXPLANATIONS

61. Provide three factors associated with wound healing and explain how these may affect the healing process.

   _____

   _____

   _____

   _____

62. Explain how the integumentary system assists in regulating body temperature.

   _____

   _____

   _____

   _____

63. List the four quadrants of the abdomen and provide at least two structures located in each of the quadrants.

   _____

   _____

   _____

   _____

64. Explain the use of the rule of nines in determining burns.

   _____

   _____

   _____

   _____

65. List three possible causes of alopecia.

   _____

   _____

   _____

   _____

66. Select five body systems and provide the major function of each one.

_____

_____

_____

_____

WHAT DO YOU DO?

67. Read the following scenario and respond to the questions with a short answer.

You are a medical assistant working in a dermatology office. Your supervisor asks you to develop a new patient education brochure on wound care. This brochure should provide instructions to patients who need to continue home care for their wound(s).

a. Write two wound care instructions that absolutely need to be included in the patient education information.

_____

_____

_____

_____

b. Write the information of signs or symptoms a patient should watch for that might indicate the wound is not healing.

_____

_____

_____

_____

c. Write the list of supplies the patient will need at home to properly care for the wound.

_____

_____

_____

_____

d. Write additional information that you would include in the patient brochure that is not included in the above items.

_____

_____

_____

_____

PATIENT EDUCATION

68. Write a short narrative script that you can use to provide patient education explaining why patients should avoid sunbathing and tanning beds.

_____

_____

_____

_____

INTERNET RESEARCH

Visit the National Institutes for Health Web site at www.nih.gov, and research the disease shingles. Provide information from this site about the cause, signs and symptoms, treatment, medication, and overall outcome of this condition. Also, include any preventive measures a person can take to avoid getting shingles.

_____

_____

_____

_____

_____

_____

_____

Chapter Objectives

- Describe the structure and growth of long bones.
- Identify the major bones of the axial skeleton.
- Identify the major bones of the appendicular skeleton.
- Describe various types of bone disorders and fractures.
- Recognize normal and abnormal curves of the spine.
- Identify the categories of joints and the movement provided by each one.
- Compare the three types of muscle tissue.
- Explain the function of skeletal muscle.
- Name some of the major muscles of the body and describe their location and function.
- Compare isotonic and isometric contractions.
- Describe major muscle disorders.
- Describe diagnostic and treatment methods associated with musculoskeletal disorders.
- Discuss the role of the medical assistant in the orthopedic office.

CAAHEP & ABHES Competencies

CAAHEP

- Describe structural organization of the human body.
- Identify body systems.
- List major organs in each body system.
- Describe the normal function of each body system.
- Identify common pathology related to each body system including signs, symptoms, and etiology.
- Analyze pathology for each body system including diagnostic measures and treatment modalities.

ABHES

- List all body systems and their structure and functions.
- Describe common diseases, symptoms, and etiologies as they apply to each system.
- Describe common diseases, diagnoses, and treatments.
- Identify diagnostic and treatment modalities as they relate to each body system.

TERMINOLOGY MATCHING

Part I Directions: Match the terms in Column A with the definitions in Column B.

Column A

1. _____ Abduction
2. _____ Adduction
3. _____ Atrophy
4. _____ Circumduction
5. _____ Dorsiflexion
6. _____ Eversion
7. _____ Extension
8. _____ Flexion
9. _____ Hyperextension
10. _____ Hypertrophy
11. _____ Insertion
12. _____ Inversion
13. _____ Isometric
14. _____ Isotonic
15. _____ Origin
16. _____ Plantar flexion
17. _____ Pronation
18. _____ Rotation
19. _____ Spasm
20. _____ Sprain
21. _____ Strain
22. _____ Supination

Column B

a. Equal or same measure, as in a muscle
b. Bending the foot downward as in standing on the tiptoes
c. Decreases the angle of the joint
d. The less moveable, fixed end of the muscle
e. Turning a bone on its own axis
f. Turning the palm of the hand down
g. Tear between the muscle and the attached tendon
h. Decrease in size or lack of development
i. Rupture or tearing of the ligaments surrounding the joint
j. Moving away from the midline of the body
k. A sudden and involuntary contraction
l. Turning the sole of the foot outward
m. Moving in a circular pattern
n. Turning the palm of the hand up
o. Moving the foot upward toward the body
p. The moveable end of the muscle attached to the bone that is moved
q. Moving toward the midline of the body
r. Increases the size or bulk of a muscle
s. Extending a body part beyond the anatomical position
t. Increases the angle of the joint
u. Equal or same tension, as in a muscle
v. Turning the sole of the foot inward

Part II Directions: Match the terms in Column A with the definitions in Column B.

Column A

23. _____ Appendicular
24. _____ Arthrocentesis
25. _____ Arthroplasty
26. _____ Arthroscopy
27. _____ Articular cartilage
28. _____ Axial
29. _____ Cancellous
30. _____ Chondrosarcoma
31. _____ Collagen
32. _____ Diaphysis
33. _____ Dislocation

34. _____ Endosteum
35. _____ Epiphyseal plates
36. _____ Fontanelles
37. _____ Ligaments
38. _____ Medullary cavity
39. _____ Osseous tissue
40. _____ Ossicles
41. _____ Ossification
42. _____ Osteoblast

Column B

a. Growth plates where continued growth of bone takes place
b. Condition with fragile, porous bones due to loss of bone mass
c. Center of the diaphysis of a long bone
d. Lining of the bone marrow cavity of a bone
e. Draining accumulated fluid from a joint cavity
f. The bones of the extremities
g. Living bone tissue
h. The cells responsible for resorption, the breakdown of bone tissue
i. Metabolic disorder known as Paget disease
j. Malignant tumor of the cartilages
k. Rare metabolic, genetic disorder resulting in defective collagen production
l. The cells responsible for building bone tissue
m. Bone infection usually caused by a pyogenic bacteria
n. Spongy bone
o. Process of cartilage converting to bone
p. Round bone found around a joint, for example, the kneecap
q. Membrane covering outside of bones
r. Form of osteomalacia that occurs in children
s. Shaft of long bones
t. Softening of the bones due to lack of calcium in the bones

43. _____ Osteoclast
44. _____ Osteocyte
45. _____ Osteogenesis imperfecta
46. _____ Osteitis deformans

47. _____ Osteomalacia
48. _____ Osteomyelitis
49. _____ Osteoporosis
50. _____ Osteosarcoma
51. _____ Periosteum
52. _____ Rickets
53. _____ Sesamoid bone
54. _____ Tendons

u. Layer of cartilage located at the ends of the bones
v. Soft spots in the infant skull
w. A protein substance that allows bones to bend slightly and not break or shatter
x. Procedure using a lighted instrument to examine the inside of a joint
y. Dense connective tissue that connects bone to bone
z. Surgical joint replacement
aa. The bones of the head and torso
bb. Dense connective tissue that attach muscles to bones
cc. Mature bone cells
dd. Tiny bones in the middle ear
ee. Structures of the joint become deranged, out of place
ff. Malignant tumor of the bone

DEFINING ABBREVIATIONS

Directions: Provide the specific meaning of each of the following abbreviations. Watch your spelling.

55. ATP: _____
_____

56. DIP: _____
_____

57. DJD: _____
_____

58. MP: _____
_____

59. PIP: _____
_____

60. OA: _____
_____

61. RA: _____
_____

MAKING IT RIGHT

Each of the following statements is false. Rewrite the statement to make it a true statement.

62. Ligaments are the structures that attach muscle to bone and tendons join bone to bone.

_____
_____
_____
_____

63. The red bone marrow produces white blood cells and the yellow marrow produces red blood cells.

_____

_____

_____

_____

64. The ribs and spinal column are part of the appendicular skeleton and the femur, tibia, humerus, and radius are part of the axial skeleton.

_____

_____

_____

_____

65. The vertebral column is composed of the 6 cervical vertebrae, 15 thoracic vertebrae, 6 lumbar vertebrae, 5 sacral bones, and 2 bones in the coccyx.

_____

_____

_____

_____

66. Osteoporosis is a condition that results in softening of the bones in children. It is due to a vitamin B deficiency.

_____

_____

_____

_____

67. Scoliosis, lordosis, and kyphosis are metabolic disorders of the skeletal system resulting in weakening of the bones of the vertebrae.

_____

_____

_____

_____

68. A greenstick fracture is a break in a bone when the bone breaks into many pieces and an impacted fracture results from a twisting of the bone.

_____

_____

_____

_____

MULTIPLE CHOICE

Directions: Choose the best answer for each question.

69. The cells responsible for building bone tissue are the:

    a. osteocytes.
    b. osteoclasts.
    c. osteoblasts.
    d. osseous cells.
    e. cancellous cells.

70. Endosteum is located in the:

    a. covering outside of the bones.
    b. ends of the bones near the joints.
    c. epiphyseal plates as the bone grows longer.
    d. inside of the bone marrow cavity.
    e. fetal skeleton prior to birth.

71. A ridge or border on a bone such as the top of the ilium is a:

    a. process.
    b. crest.
    c. foramen.
    d. sinus.
    e. fossa.

72. The bone that is located in the posterior portion of the skull is the:

    a. temporal bone.
    b. sphenoid bone.
    c. frontal bone.
    d. parietal bone.
    e. occipital bone.

73. The smaller bone of the lower leg is the:

    a. fibula.
    b. ulna.
    c. radius.
    d. tibia.
    e. patella.

74. Osteoporosis is a condition:

    a. caused by a metabolic problem due to a lack of vitamin B_{12}.
    b. occurring in children due to a lack of vitamin C.
    c. caused by a hormone imbalance.
    d. associated with fragile, porous bones.
    e. developing frequently in premenopausal women.

75. Another term for swayback is:

    a. scoliosis.
    b. kyphosis.
    c. lordosis.
    d. hunchback.
    e. porosis.

76. Which of these statements best describes a closed fracture?

    a. It is a partial break in the bone most common in children.
    b. It is a break in the bone and the broken ends become jammed into each other.
    c. It is a fracture that causes the broken part of the bone to penetrate through the skin.
    d. It is a crushing injury to a bone that does not break the skin.
    e. It is a fractured bone that does not injure the skin with an external wound.

77. Which of these is the term used for a slightly movable joint?

    a. Amphiarthrosis
    b. Synarthrosis
    c. Diarthrosis
    d. Arthrosis
    e. Osteoarthrosis

78. A fluid-filled sac found around a joint is a:

    a. synovium.
    b. bursa.
    c. cyst.
    d. disk.
    e. fossa.

79. What procedure utilizes a lighted instrument to examine a joint cavity?

    a. Osteoscopy
    b. Arthroscope
    c. Bursectomy
    d. Arthroscopy
    e. Arthrocentesis

80. What is the epimysium?

    a. It is the innermost layer that covers each muscle fiber.
    b. It is the lining of the medullary canal of a bone.
    c. It is the outermost layer that covers the entire muscle.
    d. It is the cartilage that covers the ends of bone.
    e. It is the outer layer of a developing bone.

81. A type of fracture when the bone is completely broken across the bone is a:

    a. spiral fracture.
    b. comminuted fracture.
    c. greenstick fracture.
    d. compound fracture.
    e. transverse fracture.

82. The knee joint is an example of this type of joint.

    a. Diarthrosis
    b. Amphiarthrosis
    c. Synarthrosis
    d. Fibrous
    e. Cartilaginous

83. What type of movement takes place when the foot is moved upward toward the body?

    a. Plantar flexion
    b. Abduction
    c. Hyperextension
    d. Dorsiflexion
    e. Inversion

84. The elbow and finger joints are examples of a:

    a. gliding joint.
    b. hinge joint.
    c. pivot joint.
    d. saddle joint.
    e. ball and socket joint.

85. A type of arthritis caused by an accumulation of uric acid in the joint is:

    a. rheumatoid arthritis.
    b. osteoarthritis.
    c. gouty arthritis.
    d. crippling arthritis.
    e. degenerative.

86. The physician who specializes in the treatment of musculoskeletal problems is:

    a. a physical therapist.
    b. a rheumatologist.
    c. a neurologist.
    d. an orthopedist.
    e. an occupational therapist.

87. Which one of these is a procedure used to drain fluid from a joint?

    a. Arthroplasty
    b. Arthralgia
    c. Arthroscopy
    d. Arthrotomy
    e. Arthrocentesis

88. The energy required for muscle action comes from the substance:

    a. DJD.
    b. MIP.
    c. ATP.
    d. OA.
    e. RA.

89. The main muscle that performs is the:

    a. prime mover.
    b. agonist.
    c. antagonist.
    d. voluntary muscle.
    e. contractors.

90. The dome-shaped muscle that separates the abdomen from the thorax is the:

    a. pectoralis major.
    b. rectus abdominis.
    c. intercostal muscle.
    d. diaphragm.
    e. sternocleidomastoid.

91. The major muscle of the calf is the:

    a. vastus lateralis.
    b. gastrocnemius.
    c. biceps femoris.
    d. tibialis anterior.
    e. soleus.

92. A muscle injury due to overstretching of the muscle is a:

    a. strain.
    b. sprain.
    c. cramp.
    d. spasm.
    e. tear.

93. A general term meaning pain in the muscle is:

    a. myoplegia.
    b. myositis.
    c. myalgia.
    d. myoplasty.
    e. myotonia.

BRIEF EXPLANATIONS

94. Provide three examples of bones that protect the underlying structures or organs of the body.

    _____

    _____

    _____

    _____

95. Describe the difference between the spinal curves kyphosis, lordosis, and scoliosis.

    _____

    _____

    _____

    _____

96. Provide an example of the type of body movement for each of these.

    a. Abduction - _____

    b. Adduction - _____

    c. Inversion - _____

    d. Eversion - _____

97. Explain the difference between osteoarthritis and rheumatoid arthritis.

_____

_____

_____

_____

98. Provide one example of each of these categories of bone disorders.

a. Metabolic - _____

b. Infection - _____

c. Structural - _____

d. Fracture - _____

99. Describe each of the five sections of the vertebral column including the location and number of vertebrae in the section.

_____

_____

_____

_____

WHAT DO YOU DO?

100. Read the following scenario and respond to the questions with a short answer.

Mrs. Harris, a 54-year-old woman, injured her knee while walking up stairs at her house. The physician asks you to assist with arthrocentesis of her knee. As you enter the examination room to prepare the patient, she asks what the doctor will do to her knee. She said that he really did not fully explain the procedure to her. She also wants to know why she needs to have it done for a knee injury that is just swollen. After the procedure, the physician has you complete a lab requisition to send the knee fluid for analysis. He suspects that there may be uric acid crystals in the fluid. The physician also asks you to set up an appointment with an orthopedic physician for further evaluation. She is scheduled to see the specialist, and until then, the primary physician wants her to do isotonic exercises to keep the knee strengthened.

a. Write a narrative explanation that you would provide to this patient about the arthrocentesis procedure and explain why the physician is performing it.

_____

_____

_____

_____

b. Write a narrative response to the patient about why the physician is sending the knee fluid to the laboratory for analysis.

_____

_____

_____

_____

c. How would you explain isotonic exercises that the patient needs to do until she sees the specialist?

_____

_____

_____

_____

PATIENT EDUCATION

101. The physician asks you to develop an information sheet for patients who have gout. What information do you need to include on the sheet? Research the disease and determine if there are any dietary restrictions for patients diagnosed with gout. Include this information on the information sheet.

_____

_____

_____

_____

INTERNET RESEARCH

Visit the National Institutes for Health Web site at www.nih.gov, and research the disease osteoporosis. Provide information from this site about the cause, signs and symptoms, treatment, medication, and overall outcome of this condition. Also, include any preventive measures a person can take to avoid developing osteoporosis.

_____

_____

_____

_____

_____

_____

_____

6

Nervous System, Special Senses, and Endocrine System

Chapter Objectives

- Describe the structure of a neuron.
- Describe how neuron fibers are built into a nerve.
- Explain the function of neurotransmitters in synapse transmission.
- Explain the functions of the sympathetic and parasympathetic nervous systems.
- Describe common disorders of the spinal cord and spinal nerves.
- Explain the function of the three meninges.
- Describe the function of cerebrospinal fluid.
- Identify the three subdivisions of the brain stem and the function of each.
- List the 12 cranial nerves.
- Describe disorders that affect the brain and cranial nerves.
- Explain the function of the special senses.
- Describe the major structures of the eye.
- Explain the processes involved in the sense of sight.
- Describe common disorders of the eye and vision.
- Describe the major structures of the ear.
- Explain the processes involved in the sense of hearing.
- Describe common disorders of the ear and hearing.
- Identify the glands of the endocrine system and the hormones they produce.
- Describe the functions of hormones.
- Describe common disorders of the endocrine glands.

CAAHEP & ABHES Competencies

CAAHEP

- Describe structural organization of the human body.
- Identify body systems.
- List major organs in each body system.

- Describe the normal function of each body system.
- Identify common pathology related to each body system including signs, symptoms, and etiology.
- Analyze pathology for each body system including diagnostic measures and treatment modalities.

ABHES

- List all body systems and their structure and functions.
- Describe common diseases, symptoms, and etiologies as they apply to each system.
- Identify diagnostic and treatment modalities as they relate to each body system.

TERMINOLOGY MATCHING

Part I Directions: Match the terms in Column A with the definitions in Column B.

Column A

1. _____ Acromegaly
2. _____ Axons
3. _____ Cataract
4. _____ Cerebrum
5. _____ Ceruminosis
6. _____ Conjunctivitis
7. _____ Dendrites
8. _____ Diabetes mellitus
9. _____ Epinephrine
10. _____ Gigantism
11. _____ Glaucoma
12. _____ Incus
13. _____ Malleus
14. _____ Meninges
15. _____ Myelin
16. _____ Myopia
17. _____ Nerve
18. _____ Neurons
19. _____ Neuropathy
20. _____ Otitis media
21. _____ Paraplegia
22. _____ Poliomyelitis
23. _____ Quadriplegia
24. _____ Reflex
25. _____ Sciatica
26. _____ Seizure
27. _____ Stapes
28. _____ Synapse

Column B

a. Composed of a bundle of neuron fibers
b. Hammer-shaped bone in the middle ear
c. Paralysis of all four limbs
d. Compression of a nerve of the lower back causing pain, numbness, and tingling from the lower back continuing down the leg
e. Abnormal electrical activity in the brain, which causes uncontrollable muscle contractions
f. Whitish, fatty substance that covers some of the axons just like insulation
g. Allows transmission of the impulse from the axon of one neuron to the dendrite of another neuron
h. An involuntary response to a stimulus
i. Neuron fibers that conduct impulses *to* the cell body
j. Cloudiness of the lens causing gradual loss of vision
k. Largest part of the brain divided into a right and left hemisphere
l. Overproduction of the growth hormone causing enlargement of extremities in adults
m. Nearsightedness
n. Inflammation of the conjunctiva
o. Paralysis of both lower limbs
p. Stirrup-shaped bone in the middle ear
q. Causes a child to grow abnormally tall
r. Impacted ear wax
s. Elevated glucose in the blood, a result of insulin deficiency
t. Excessive pressure of the aqueous humor
u. Coverings that surround and protect the brain and spinal cord
v. Neuron fibers that conduct impulses away from the cell body
w. Anvil-shaped bone in the middle ear
x. Highly specialized cells of the nervous system
y. Known as adrenaline, primary hormone produced in the adrenal medulla
z. A viral disease of the nervous system
aa. Infection and inflammation of the middle ear
bb. Any disease of the nervous system

DEFINING ABBREVIATIONS

Directions: Provide the specific meaning of each of the following abbreviations. Watch your spelling.

29. ACTH: _____

_____

30. ADH: _____

_____

31. ALS: _____

_____

32. CNS: _____

_____

33. CSF: _____

_____

34. CT: _____

_____

35. CVA: _____

_____

36. EEG: _____

_____

37. FSH: _____

_____

38. GH: _____

_____

39. LH: _____

_____

40. MRI: _____

_____

41. MS: _____

_____

42. MTBI: _____

_____

43. PET: _____

_____

44. PNS: _____

_____

45. T1DM: _____

_____

46. T2DM: _____

_____

47. TSH: _____

_____

MAKING IT RIGHT

Each of the following statements is false. Rewrite the statement to make it a true statement.

48. The peripheral nervous system divides into the central nervous system and the visceral nervous system.

_____

_____

_____

_____

49. Efferent neurons are the sensory neurons and afferent neurons are the motor neurons.

_____

_____

_____

_____

50. The sympathetic nervous system slows the heart rate and the parasympathetic nervous system increases the rate and force of the heart contractions.

_____

_____

_____

_____

51. Sciatica causes a partial facial paralysis due to inflammation of the VII facial nerve.

_____

_____

_____

_____

52. Meningitis is associated with a disorder of the nervous system caused from a virus that lies dormant along a nerve. It causes nerve pain and a severe skin rash.

_____

_____

_____

_____

53. A cataract is an eye condition caused from inflammation of the conjunctiva due to an irritant or pathogen.

_____

_____

_____

_____

54. Hyperopia, farsightedness, is a condition that affects a person's vision causing them to see things close to them but not far away.

_____

_____

_____

_____

MULTIPLE CHOICE

Directions: Choose the best answer for each question.

55. The autonomic nervous system is also known as the:

    a. voluntary nervous system.
    b. central nervous system.
    c. effector nervous system.
    d. somatic nervous system.
    e. visceral nervous system.

56. The whitish, fatty substance that covers some of the axons is the:

    a. meninges.
    b. neuron.
    c. myelin.
    d. synapse.
    e. interneuron.

57. How many pair of spinal nerves branch off the spinal cord?

    a. 15
    b. 21
    c. 25
    d. 31
    e. 35

58. The knee–jerk response is an example of a:

    a. voluntary reaction.
    b. reflex.
    c. synapse.
    d. stimulus.
    e. nerve message.

59. The nerve that carries visual impulses from the eye to the brain is the:

    a. trochlear nerve.
    b. trigeminal nerve.
    c. optic nerve.
    d. oculomotor nerve.
    e. facial nerve.

60. The midbrain, pons, and medulla oblongata are located in the:

    a. brain stem.
    b. diencephalon.
    c. hypothalamus.
    d. cerebellum.
    e. cerebrum.

61. An invasive procedure that involves inserting a needle into the space between vertebrae to withdraw a small amount of CSF is a:

    a. thoracocentesis.
    b. spinoplasty.
    c. laminectomy.
    d. myelonectomy.
    e. lumbar puncture.

62. Paralysis of both lower limbs is:

    a. monoplegia.
    b. hemiplegia.
    c. paraplegia.
    d. bilateral paralysis.
    e. quadriplegia.

63. Encephalitis is inflammation of the:

    a. brain.
    b. spinal cord.
    c. meninges.
    d. vertebrae and spinal cord.
    e. cerebrospinal fluid.

64. A progressive neurologic condition causing tremors and rigidity of the limbs and joints is:

    a. hydrocephalus.
    b. Alzheimer disease.
    c. Parkinson disease.
    d. sciatica.
    e. traumatic brain disease.

65. A cerebrovascular accident is due to a:

    a. concussion.
    b. blood clot.
    c. bacterial infection.
    d. seizure disorder.
    e. spinal injury.

66. What structure of the eye is the window of the eye?

   a. Choroid
   b. Cornea
   c. Iris
   d. Pupil
   e. Sclera

67. Deterioration of the fovea centralis region on the retina causes:

   a. cataracts.
   b. glaucoma.
   c. myopia.
   d. retinopathy.
   e. macular degeneration.

68. Strabismus is an eye condition that causes:

   a. distorted lenses.
   b. corneal abrasion.
   c. farsightedness.
   d. crossed eyes.
   e. nearsightedness.

69. The medical doctor who specializes in the treatment of eye conditions and performs eye surgery is an:

   a. optician.
   b. optometrist.
   c. oculist.
   d. optical technologist.
   e. ophthalmologist.

70. The structure that connects the middle ear with the throat is the:

   a. eustachian tube.
   b. external auditory canal.
   c. tympanic tube.
   d. semicircular canal.
   e. vestibule.

71. Otitis externa is also known as:

   a. presbycusis.
   b. otosclerosis.
   c. swimmer's ear.
   d. tympanitis.
   e. vertigo.

72. The master gland of the endocrine system is the:

   a. thyroid.
   b. pituitary.
   c. adrenal.
   d. pancreas.
   e. thymus.

73. The hormone that stimulates milk production in the breasts is:

    a. ACTH.
    b. FSH.
    c. LH.
    d. PRL.
    e. ADH.

74. The endocrine gland that secretes a hormone promoting calcium release from bone tissue into the blood is the:

    a. adrenal gland.
    b. pancreas.
    c. parathyroid gland.
    d. thyroid gland.
    e. posterior pituitary.

75. Which gland secretes the hormone epinephrine?

    a. Adrenal medulla
    b. Adrenal cortex
    c. Anterior pituitary
    d. Posterior pituitary
    e. Hypothalamus

76. The islets of Langerhans are located in the:

    a. adrenal cortex.
    b. thymus gland.
    c. parathyroid glands.
    d. hypothalamus.
    e. pancreas.

77. The primary hormone responsible for the development of secondary female sex characteristics is:

    a. progesterone.
    b. estrogen.
    c. luteinizing hormone.
    d. prolactin.
    e. oxytocin.

78. The gland that has both exocrine and endocrine function is the:

    a. adrenal gland.
    b. pituitary gland.
    c. pancreas.
    d. thymus.
    e. thyroid gland.

79. Graves disease causes the development of:

    a. diabetes.
    b. extremity enlargement.
    c. kidney stones.
    d. goiter.
    e. excessive skin pigmentation.

BRIEF EXPLANATIONS

80. Explain the functions of cerebrospinal fluid and the purpose of performing a lumbar puncture.

_____

_____

_____

_____

81. Explain what specifically happens that causes a knee–jerk response.

_____

_____

_____

_____

82. Provide an explanation of how the sympathetic and parasympathetic systems perform opposing actions for these body structures or functions.

a. Heart rate - _____

b. Bronchial tubes - _____

83. Explain the function of each of these special sense receptors.

a. Chemoreceptors - _____

b. Photoreceptors - _____

c. Thermoreceptors - _____

d. Mechanoreceptors - _____

84. Describe how each of these structures protect the eye.

a. Eyelashes and eyebrows - _____

b. Lacrimal glands - _____

c. Conjunctiva - _____

WHAT DO YOU DO?

85. Read the following scenario and respond to the questions with a short answer.

Paula Summers, a 36-year-old patient, is in the office as a follow-up from a visit to the emergency department, over the weekend. She had a strep throat infection and a high fever. She also experienced a seizure. The office physician asks you to schedule her for an EEG to rule out underlying problems related to the seizure episode.

a. Write a narrative explanation that helps the patient to understand the reason for performing the EEG and what the physician means by underlying problems. Provide an example in your explanation.

_____

_____

_____

_____

b. How will you respond to the patient if she asks if she has epilepsy since she thinks epilepsy is the only cause for all seizures?

_____

_____

_____

_____

c. The patient asks you what actually happens when you have a seizure. How would you explain this to her?

_____

_____

_____

_____

PATIENT EDUCATION

86. The physician asks you to develop an information sheet for parents to encourage them to vaccinate their children with the polio vaccine. What information should be included that will impress the importance of this vaccination?

_____

_____

_____

_____

INTERNET RESEARCH

Visit the National Institutes for Health Web site at www.nih.gov, and research the condition of stroke, cerebrovascular accident. Provide information about the cause, signs and symptoms, treatment, medication, and overall outcome of this condition. Also, include any preventive measures a person can take to avoid having a stroke.

_____

_____

_____

_____

_____

_____

_____

7 Digestive System and Nutrition

Chapter Objectives

- Describe the function of the digestive system.
- List the organs of the digestive tract and describe their specific function.
- List the accessory organs of digestion and describe how they assist the digestive system.
- Explain the process of absorption in the digestive system.
- Explain the purpose of bile.
- Describe the muscular contraction of the digestive system.
- Describe common disorders of the digestive tract and the accessory organs.
- Describe the roles of minerals and vitamins in the body.
- Explain the use of protein, carbohydrates, and fats in the body.
- Compare saturated and unsaturated fats.
- Describe common nutritional disorders.

CAAHEP & ABHES Competencies

CAAHEP

- Describe structural organization of the human body.
- Identify body systems.
- List major organs in each body system.
- Describe the normal function of each body system.
- Identify common pathology related to each body system including signs, symptoms, and etiology.
- Analyze pathology for each body system including diagnostic measures and treatment modalities.

ABHES

- List all body systems and their structure and functions.
- Describe common diseases, symptoms, and etiologies as they apply to each system.
- Identify diagnostic and treatment modalities as they relate to each body system.

TERMINOLOGY MATCHING

Part I Directions: Match the terms in Column A with the definitions in Column B.

Column A

1. _____ Anorexia
2. _____ Appendicitis
3. _____ Chyme
4. _____ Cholecystectomy
5. _____ Cholelithiasis
6. _____ Cirrhosis
7. _____ Defecation
8. _____ Diverticulosis
9. _____ Endoscopy
10. _____ Gastritis
11. _____ Hepatitis
12. _____ Ingestion
13. _____ Mastication
14. _____ Nausea
15. _____ Oral thrush
16. _____ Parotitis
17. _____ Peristalsis
18. _____ Ulcerative colitis
19. _____ Villi
20. _____ Vomiting

Column B

a. Feeling of queasiness that usually precedes vomiting
b. Finger-like projections found on the mucosal lining of the small intestine
c. Formation of gallstones that may block the bile ducts
d. Process of chewing the food
e. Yeast infection in the mouth
f. Inflammation and ulceration of the colon and rectum
g. Surgical removal of the gallbladder
h. Semiliquid substance that moves from the stomach to the duodenum
i. Inflammation of the parotid glands
j. Inflammation of the appendix due to infection or obstruction
k. Rhythmic action of moving material through the large intestine
l. Chronic liver disease
m. Process of expelling the stomach contents through the mouth
n. Inflammation of the liver
o. Chronic loss of appetite
p. Small pouches in the wall of the intestine
q. Process of eliminating the waste from the body
r. Process of taking food into the mouth
s. Inflammation of the stomach lining
t. Use of a lighted scope to visualize the gastrointestinal tract

DEFINING ABBREVIATIONS

Directions: Provide the specific meaning of each of the following abbreviations. Watch your spelling.

21. BMR: _____

_____

22. GERD: _____

_____

23. GI: _____

_____

24. HBV: _____

_____

25. HCL: _____

_____

26. IBD: _____

_____

27. IBS: _____

_____

28. LES: _____

_____

29. LDL: _____

_____

MAKING IT RIGHT

Each of the following statements is false. Rewrite the statement to make it a true statement.

30. The sublingual glands are at the back of the mouth in front of the ear and become inflamed when someone has the mumps.

_____

_____

_____

_____

31. Cholelithiasis is a surgical removal of the gallbladder due to excessive stone formation.

_____

_____

_____

_____

32. Diverticulosis is the development of a large number of varicose veins of the rectum.

_____

_____

_____

_____

33. Nausea and vomiting are diseases of the stomach that only occur during infectious conditions in the body.

_____

_____

_____

_____

34. The sunshine vitamin is vitamin C and vitamin K is necessary to help the body absorb calcium.

_____

_____

_____

_____

35. The two layers of the peritoneum are the parietal peritoneum that covers the abdominal organs and the visceral peritoneum that lines the wall of the abdominal cavity.

_____

_____

_____

_____

36. The salivary glands include the sublingual gland located beneath the mandible, the parotid gland located under the tongue, and the submandibular located under the tongue.

_____

_____

_____

_____

MULTIPLE CHOICE

Directions: Choose the best answer for each question.

37. The other name for the cardiac sphincter is the:

    a. pyloric sphincter.
    b. ileocecal sphincter.
    c. lower esophageal sphincter.
    d. hiatal sphincter.
    e. upper visceral sphincter.

38. The strong acid in the stomach is:

    a. HCL.
    b. LDL.
    c. IBD.
    d. IBD.
    e. HBV.

39. The portion of the pharynx visible when the mouth is open is the:

    a. esophagopharynx.
    b. laryngopharynx.
    c. oropharynx.
    d. nasopharynx.
    e. gingivopharynx.

40. The uppermost rounded part of the stomach is the:

    a. pylorus.
    b. hiatus.
    c. lesser curvature.
    d. body.
    e. fundus.

41. The substance that leaves the stomach to enter the small intestine is:

   a. a bolus.
   b. pepsin.
   c. optic nerve.
   d. chyme.
   e. gastric juice.

42. The middle part of the small intestine is the:

   a. ileum.
   b. jejunum.
   c. sigmoid.
   d. duodenum.
   e. pylorus.

43. Which of these are finger-like projections located on the mucosal lining of the small intestine?

   a. Rugae
   b. Diverticuli
   c. Varicosities
   d. Villi
   e. Valves

44. The portion of the colon that extends from the cecum on the right side of the abdomen is the:

   a. ascending colon.
   b. descending colon.
   c. transverse colon.
   d. ileocecal colon.
   e. sigmoid colon.

45. Bacteria, normally found in the colon, produce vitamin:

   a. A.
   b. C.
   c. D.
   d. E.
   e. K.

46. The largest accessory organ in the digestive system is the:

   a. pancreas.
   b. liver.
   c. gallbladder.
   d. spleen.
   e. stomach.

47. The substance that gives color to stool is:

   a. hydrochloric acid.
   b. bile.
   c. pancreatic juice.
   d. bilirubin.
   e. vitamin K.

48. What is the function of bile?

    a. Digest carbohydrates
    b. Breakdown fats
    c. Produce vitamin K
    d. Destroys old red blood cells
    e. Metabolize drugs

49. Which of these causes decreased activity in the digestive tract?

    a. Parasympathetic nervous system
    b. Peristalsis in the small intestine
    c. Sympathetic nervous system
    d. Endocrine action of the pancreas
    e. Release of sodium bicarbonate from the pancreas

50. The regulation of the sensation of hunger occurs in the:

    a. hypothalamus.
    b. stomach.
    c. salivary glands.
    d. cerebellum.
    e. small intestine.

51. The height and weight of a person to determine the body fat is the:

    a. body fat content.
    b. body adipose content.
    c. body mass index.
    d. base fat content.
    e. base mass index.

52. Which of these is the condition when a person eats food then forces vomiting
    to get the food out before digesting and absorbing it?

    a. Appetite suppression
    b. Appetite control
    c. Bulimia
    d. Fasting
    e. Starving

53. Which agency developed the Choose MyPlate?

    a. ADA
    b. EPA
    c. CDC
    d. WHO
    e. USDA

54. Which of these conditions results from a serious shortage of protein in the
    diet?

    a. Pancreatitis
    b. Anorexia
    c. Bulimia
    d. Kwashiorkor
    e. Rickets

55. Which of these is the condition of developing gallstones?

    a. Cholecystitis
    b. Cholelithiasis
    c. Cholecystectomy
    d. Colitis
    e. Cholitis

56. Hepatitis A transmission is primarily through:

    a. contaminated food and water.
    b. coughing and sneezing.
    c. contaminated needles.
    d. infected blood.
    e. sexual contact.

57. The common cause of cirrhosis of the liver is:

    a. consuming a high-fat diet.
    b. excessive alcohol consumption.
    c. overuse of anti-inflammatory drugs.
    d. overproduction of bile.
    e. extreme dieting.

58. Which of these procedures uses a lighted scope to visualize the colon?

    a. Cholecystoscopy
    b. Gastroscopy
    c. Hepatoscopy
    d. Colonoscopy
    e. Duodenoscopy

59. Varicosed veins of the rectum are:

    a. polyps.
    b. diverticuli.
    c. hemorrhoids.
    d. rugae.
    e. cysts.

60. Which of these is a condition when a person cannot tolerate gluten in their diet?

    a. Crohn disease
    b. Cholecystitis
    c. Ulcerative colitis
    d. Irritable bowel syndrome
    e. Celiac disease

61. Which bacteria found in the stomach stimulates the production of HCL?

    a. *Mycobacterium ulcerans*
    b. *Streptococcus pyogenes*
    c. *Escherichia coli*
    d. *Helicobacter pylori*
    e. *Haemophilus influenzae*

BRIEF EXPLANATIONS

62. Explain the structure and function of the esophagus including any changes it makes to the food we eat.

_____

_____

_____

_____

63. Explain the purpose of the rugae in the stomach.

_____

_____

_____

_____

64. Explain the purpose of these accessory organs of the digestive system.

   a. Liver - _____

   b. Gallbladder - _____

   c. Pancreas - _____

65. Explain the difference between ingestion, digestion, and absorption.

_____

_____

_____

_____

66. List four (4) functions of the liver.

   a. _____

   b. _____

   c. _____

   d. _____

WHAT DO YOU DO?

67. Read the following scenario and respond to the questions with a short answer.

The physician sees Mark Summers, a 48-year-old patient, who is experiencing chest pain. The physician does not believe that this problem is heart related. He asks you to schedule the patient to see a gastroenterologist for further evaluation.

a. Write a narrative explanation that helps the patient understand the reason for seeing the stomach specialist.

_____

_____

_____

_____

b. How will you respond to the patient if he asks why he is having chest pain but no heart-related problem?

_____

_____

_____

_____

PATIENT EDUCATION

68. The physician asks you to develop an information sheet for patients who need to improve their diet. What information should be included about the importance of protein, carbohydrates, and fats in the diet?

_____

_____

_____

_____

INTERNET RESEARCH

Visit the National Institutes for Health Web site at www.nih.gov, and research the condition of anorexia nervosa. Provide information about the cause, signs and symptoms, treatment, medication, and overall outcome of this condition. Include the negative effects of this condition on the body.

_____

_____

_____

_____

_____

_____

_____

Cardiovascular and Respiratory Systems

Chapter Objectives

- Describe the function of the cardiovascular system.
- Describe the chambers of the heart and their function.
- Describe the location and function of the valves of the heart.
- Describe the three tissue layers of the heart wall.
- List the structures of the vascular system.
- Briefly describe blood circulation through the myocardium.
- Describe the cardiac cycle.
- Name and locate the components of the heart's conduction system.
- Define common terms that describe variations in heart rates.
- Identify common types of heart disease.
- List risk factors for coronary artery disease.
- List common diagnostic exams used to detect cardiovascular disorders.
- Describe common approaches to the treatment of heart disease.
- List the different types of blood vessels.
- List common disorders of the circulatory system.
- Explain the process of respiration and the factors that control respiration.
- Name and describe all the structures of the respiratory system.
- Discuss the processes of internal and external gas exchange.
- Explain the process for the transportation of oxygen and carbon dioxide in the blood.
- List common types of respiratory disorders.
- List the common procedures and treatments used for respiratory diseases.

CAAHEP & ABHES Competencies

CAAHEP

- Describe structural organization of the human body.
- Identify body systems.

● List major organs in each body system.
● Describe the normal function of each body system.
● Identify common pathology related to each body system including signs, symptoms, and etiology.
● Analyze pathology for each body system including diagnostic measures and treatment modalities.

ABHES

● List all body systems and their structure and functions.
● Describe common diseases, symptoms, and etiologies as they apply to each system.
● Identify diagnostic and treatment modalities as they relate to each body system.

TERMINOLOGY MATCHING

Part I Directions: Match the terms in Column A with the definitions in Column B.

Column A

1. _____ Aneurysm
2. _____ Apex
3. _____ Arrhythmia

4. _____ Arteriosclerosis
5. _____ Atherosclerosis
6. _____ Atrioventricular
7. _____ Bradycardia
8. _____ Bronchodilators

9. _____ Bronchoscope
10. _____ Carbaminohemoglobin

11. _____ Cardiologist
12. _____ Catheterization
13. _____ Coronary angiography
14. _____ Coronary
15. _____ Deoxygenated
16. _____ Diastole
17. _____ Dysrhythmia

18. _____ Endocarditis
19. _____ Endocardium
20. _____ Effusion
21. _____ Epicardium
22. _____ Epistaxis
23. _____ Hypertension
24. _____ Hypotension
25. _____ Ischemia

26. _____ Mediastinum
27. _____ Murmur

28. _____ Myocarditis
29. _____ Myocardium

Column B

a. In the central area of the chest cavity
b. Active, contracting phase of the heart
c. Term that means a crown, which is how the vessels encircle the heart
d. A heart specialist
e. Inflammation of the sac around the heart
f. Used to describe an abnormal heart rhythm, same as dysrhythmia
g. High blood pressure
h. An invasive procedure used to diagnose or treat conditions affecting circulation in the coronary arteries
i. Accumulation of fluid as a result of fluid leaking into a space
j. The outermost layer of the heart, which also serves as the visceral layer of the pericardium
k. Rapid heart rate of more than 100 bpm
l. Lower, rounded area of the heart
m. Slow heart rate of less than 60 bpm
n. Caused by a faulty heart valve that fails to close tightly
o. Blood that has less oxygen
p. Condition caused by a buildup of plaque
q. Dye is injected into the coronary arteries to highlight any vessel damage or blockage
r. Blood that is rich in oxygen
s. Inflammation of the heart muscle
t. A fibrous sac surrounding the heart
u. A normal heart rhythm
v. Pertaining to the atria and ventricles
w. Half moon shape as some of the valves in the heart
x. Oxygen binding with hemoglobin
y. Bulging or ballooning sac of a vessel due to weakness in the wall of the vessel
z. Resting, relaxing phase of the heart
aa. The innermost lining of the heart covering the inside of the heart chambers and heart valves
bb. Lack of blood supply
cc. Used to describe an abnormal heart rhythm, same as arrhythmia

30. _____ Necrosis
31. _____ Oxygenated
32. _____ Oxyhemoglobin
33. _____ Pericarditis
34. _____ Pericardium
35. _____ Plaque
36. _____ -pnea

37. _____ Semilunar
38. _____ Sinus rhythm
39. _____ Spirometer
40. _____ Stenosis
41. _____ Systole
42. _____ Tachycardia
43. _____ Thrombosis

dd. Blood clot formation
ee. Narrowing of the valve opening
ff. Low blood pressure
gg. Instrument used to visually examine the inside of the lungs
hh. Carbon dioxide combined with hemoglobin
ii. Nosebleed
jj. Hardening of the arteries caused by loss of elasticity of the arterial wall
kk. The muscular layer of the heart, cardiac muscle
ll. Device used to test a patient's breathing
mm. Fatty deposits
nn. Inflammation of the inside lining of the heart
oo. Death of tissue
pp. Word root that refers to breathing
qq. Used to relax and dilate the bronchioles of the lungs

DEFINING ABBREVIATIONS

Directions: Provide the specific meaning of each of the following abbreviations. Watch your spelling.

44. ARDS: _____

_____

45. AV: _____

_____

46. bpm: _____

_____

47. CABG: _____

_____

48. COPD: _____

_____

49. CO_2: _____

_____

50. CPR: _____

_____

51. CT: _____

_____

52. ECG/EKG: _____

_____

53. MI: _____

_____

54. NSR: _____

_____

55. O₂: _____

_____

56. PAC: _____

_____

57. PAT: _____

_____

58. PTCA: _____

_____

59. PVC: _____

_____

60. RSV: _____

_____

61. SA: _____

_____

62. TB: _____

_____

63. URI: _____

_____

MAKING IT RIGHT

Each of the following statements is false. Rewrite the statement to make it a true statement.

64. The right atrium receives oxygenated blood from the lungs and the left ventricle receives blood from the body and pumps it to the lungs to oxygenate.

_____

_____

_____

65. Another name for the bundle of His is the atrioventricular node.

_____

_____

_____

66. Sinus bradycardia is an abnormally rapid heartbeat resulting in decreased ventricular filling and low blood pressure.

_____

_____

_____

_____

67. Atherosclerosis is a condition caused by a lack of blood supply to the heart muscle.

_____

_____

_____

_____

68. Anticoagulants are medications that reduce the rate and strength of heart contractions.

_____

_____

_____

_____

69. An aneurysm is caused from the formation of a blood clot in a blood vessel.

_____

_____

_____

_____

MULTIPLE CHOICE

Directions: Choose the best answer for each question.

70. Swollen, gnarled veins that do not work effectively to move blood are:

    a. sclerosed.
    b. narrowed.
    c. varicosed.
    d. ruptured.
    e. oxygenated.

71. The heart valve that is between the left atrium and left ventricle is the:

    a. aortic valve.
    b. mitral valve.
    c. tricuspid valve.
    d. coronary valve.
    e. pulmonary valve.

72. On the ECG tracing, the contraction of the ventricles is represented by the:

    a. P wave.
    b. QRS complex.
    c. PR interval.
    d. T wave.
    e. ST segment.

73. Which of these is the term for inflammation of the heart muscle?

    a. Epicarditis
    b. Endocarditis
    c. Pericarditis
    d. Myocarditis
    e. Vasculitis

74. An abnormally slow heartbeat but with a normal rhythm is:

    a. atrial flutter.
    b. normal sinus rhythm.
    c. a premature ventricular contraction.
    d. paroxysmal atrial tachycardia.
    e. sinus bradycardia.

75. Which of these is a congenital condition?

    a. Mitral valve prolapse
    b. Endocarditis
    c. Tetralogy of Fallot
    d. Arteriosclerosis
    e. Atherosclerosis

76. Which of these is a medication a patient would take during angina pectoris to help open the coronary vessels?

    a. Nitroglycerin
    b. Beta-blocker
    c. Penicillin
    d. Bronchodilator
    e. Anticoagulant

77. What is the major cause of developing COPD?

    a. Cigarette smoking
    b. Strep infections
    c. Chemical fumes
    d. Pollen
    e. Allergies

78. Which of these is an accumulation of air in the pleural space?

    a. Pyothorax
    b. Hemothorax
    c. Pleurisy
    d. Atelectasis
    e. Pneumothorax

79. Which of these treats bacterial infections in the lungs?

    a. Analgesics
    b. Antibiotics
    c. Bronchodilators
    d. Steroids
    e. Vasodilators

80. Which of these components of the ECG tracing represents the resting period of the heart before the next cardiac cycle begins?

    a. P wave
    b. R wave
    c. ST segment
    d. T wave
    e. QRS complex

81. Which of these represents the correct sequence of electrical activity in the heart?

    a. AV node to the Purkinje fibers
    b. AV node to the SA node
    c. SA node to the AV node
    d. Bundle of His to the AV node
    e. Bundle branches to the bundle of His

82. The semilunar valve that allows blood flow from the right ventricle into the pulmonary blood vessels leading to the lungs is the:

    a. aortic valve.
    b. pulmonary valve.
    c. mitral valve.
    d. bicuspid valve.
    e. tricuspid valve.

83. A heartbeat of 40 bpm is:

    a. caused by a heart murmur.
    b. classified as bradycardia.
    c. due to narrowing of a valve.
    d. classified as fibrillation.
    e. classified as tachycardia.

84. PVC is:

    a. a congenital problem.
    b. caused by a defect in the SA node.
    c. a premature contraction of the ventricle.
    d. a serious infection in the heart.
    e. the same as a defective heart valve.

85. Endocarditis involves the:

    a. inside lining of the heart.
    b. sac around the heart.
    c. coronary arteries.
    d. outer lining of the heart.
    e. pulmonary vessels.

86. Which of these procedures records the electrical activity of the heart?

    a. Catheterization
    b. Echocardiogram
    c. Angiography
    d. Computerized tomography
    e. Electrocardiogram

87. Which infection is caused by a bacillus type of bacteria?

    a. Asthma
    b. Bronchitis
    c. Tuberculosis
    d. Emphysema
    e. Atelectasis

88. Surfactant is:

    a. a substance that increases the heart rate.
    b. used to treat asthma.
    c. an anti-inflammatory.
    d. the substance that facilitates lung expansion.
    e. found in the heart chambers to keep the valves functioning.

89. Another term for a sore throat is:

    a. laryngitis.
    b. pharyngitis.
    c. rhinitis.
    d. sinusitis.
    e. esophagitis.
    f. extreme dieting.

BRIEF EXPLANATIONS

90. Explain the difference between a pneumothorax and hemothorax.

    _____

    _____

    _____

    _____

91. Explain the function of the alveoli in the lungs.

    _____

    _____

    _____

    _____

92. Explain each of these terms for types of breathing.

    a. Apnea: _____

    b. Dyspnea: _____

    c. Orthopnea: _____

WHAT DO YOU DO?

93. Read the following scenario and respond to the questions with a short answer.

Mrs. Masters was in the emergency room over the weekend for chest discomfort with shortness of breath. Your physician examined her and asked you to do an electrocardiogram. When the physician reviews the ECG, he informs the patient that there are a couple of concerns with the tracing and wants her to be further evaluated by a cardiologist.

a. Write a narrative explanation that helps the patient understand the reason for seeing the cardiologist.

_____

_____

_____

_____

b. How will you respond to the patient if asked what the doctor meant by "couple of concerns on the tracing"?

_____

_____

_____

_____

PATIENT EDUCATION

94. The physician asks you to develop an information sheet for patients who have cardiac conditions. What signs and symptoms are important to include in the sheet that patients should be aware of and concerned about?

_____

_____

_____

_____

INTERNET RESEARCH

Visit the National Institutes for Health Web site at www.nih.gov and research the condition of cardiomyopathy. Provide information about the cause, signs and symptoms, treatment, medication, and overall outcome of this condition. Include the negative effects of this condition on the body.

_____

_____

_____

_____

_____

_____

_____

9 Urinary and Reproductive Systems

Chapter Objectives

- List the urinary system organs and the function of each.
- Explain the kidney's role in maintaining homeostasis.
- Describe the function of the nephron.
- Explain the process of urine formation.
- Explain the process of urination.
- Discuss various types of urinary system disorders.
- Explain the purpose of renal dialysis.
- List the organs of the male and female reproductive systems.
- Describe the function of the male and female reproductive organs.
- Describe a spermatozoon and describe the function of semen.
- Identify the hormones that regulate the male and female reproductive organs.
- Discuss various types of male and female reproductive system disorders.
- Explain the changes during and after menopause.
- Describe the process of fertilization.
- Explain the main process of fetal development.
- List the stages of labor.

CAAHEP & ABHES Competencies

CAAHEP

- Describe structural organization of the human body.
- Identify body systems.
- List major organs in each body system.
- Describe the normal function of each body system.
- Identify common pathology related to each body system including signs, symptoms, and etiology.
- Analyze pathology for each body system including diagnostic measures and treatment modalities.

ABHES

- List all body systems and their structure and functions.
- Describe common diseases, symptoms, and etiologies as they apply to each system.
- Identify diagnostic and treatment modalities as they relate to each body system.

TERMINOLOGY MATCHING

Part I Directions: Match the terms in Column A with the definitions in Column B.

Column A

1. _____ Abortion
2. _____ Cesarean section
3. _____ Cryptorchidism
4. _____ Cystitis
5. _____ Dialysis

6. _____ Dysmenorrhea
7. _____ Endometriosis
8. _____ Endometrium
9. _____ Enuresis
10. _____ Episiotomy
11. _____ Excretory

12. _____ Glomerulonephritis
13. _____ Glycosuria
14. _____ Hematuria

15. _____ Hydronephrosis
16. _____ Incontinence
17. _____ Lithotripsy

18. _____ Mammogram
19. _____ Micturition
20. _____ Ovulation
21. _____ Pyelonephritis
22. _____ Pyuria

23. _____ Uremia

24. _____ Ureterocele
25. _____ Urethritis

Column B

a. Pus in the urine
b. Type of herniation of the ureter as it enters the bladder
c. Condition when the endometrial tissue grows outside the uterus
d. Inflammation of the renal pelvis
e. A small incision between the vagina and the anus to increase the size of the delivery area
f. An x-ray study of the breast to detect growths
g. Blood in the urine
h. Involuntary loss of urine
i. Process of releasing an egg from the ovary follicle
j. Accumulation of fluid in the kidney
k. Use of a machine to filter the blood when the kidneys are unable to work properly
l. Inflammation of the urethra
m. Excess of nitrogen waste substances in the blood
n. Inflammation of the bladder due to infection and retention of urine in the bladder
o. Involuntary urination usually occurring at night (bedwetting)
p. Inner lining of the uterus
q. Damage to the glomerulus and kidney usually as response to strep infection
r. Glucose in the urine
s. Painful or difficult menstruation
t. Procedure to crush kidney stones
u. Another term used to describe the urinary system
v. General term that means the loss of the embryo or fetus prior to week 20 of a pregnancy
w. A surgical incision made in the abdominal wall and uterus to deliver a baby
x. Undescended testicle
y. The process of urination

DEFINING ABBREVIATIONS

Directions: Provide the specific meaning of each of the following abbreviations. Watch your spelling.

26. ADH: _____

_____

27. BPH: _____

_____

28. EDC: _____

_____

29. ESWL: _____

_____

30. FSH: _____

_____

31. HPV: _____

_____

32. HRT: _____

_____

33. LH: _____

_____

34. LMP: _____

_____

35. PID: _____

_____

36. PMS: _____

_____

37. PSA: _____

_____

38. STI: _____

_____

39. TAH: _____

_____

40. UTI: _____

_____

MAKING IT RIGHT

Each of the following statements is false. Rewrite the statement to make it a true statement.

41. The ureter is the urinary tube that leads from the bladder to the outside of the body.

_____

_____

_____

_____

42. The hormone LH is released by the posterior pituitary gland and controls the reabsorption of water.

_____

_____

_____

_____

43. A ureterocele is a condition in the male where the urethral opening is on the underside of the penis instead of the end of the penis.

_____

_____

_____

_____

44. Acute renal failure is a genetic disorder resulting in development of fluid-filled sacs in the kidney.

_____

_____

_____

_____

45. Phimosis is an undescended testicle that could result in infertility if uncorrected.

_____

_____

_____

_____

46. The myometrium is the layer of the uterus that prepares to receive a fertilized egg.

_____

_____

_____

_____

MULTIPLE CHOICE

Directions: Choose the best answer for each question.

47. The kidneys are located:

    a. in the lower lumbar region of the back.
    b. in the pelvic cavity.
    c. behind the peritoneum at the level of the lower thoracic and upper lumbar region.
    d. by the urinary bladder in the hypogastric region of the abdomen.
    e. below the liver in the peritoneal cavity.

48. What structure is supplied with blood from the afferent arteriole and leaves through the efferent arteriole?

    a. Loop of Henle
    b. Descending tubule
    c. Renal pelvis
    d. Glomerulus
    e. Renal cortex

49. The approximate amount of urine produced each day is:

    a. 1.5 to 2 L.
    b. 4 to 5 L.
    c. 8 to 10 L.
    d. 12 to 15 L.
    e. 15 to 20 L.

50. The hormone that controls the reabsorption of water in the kidneys is:

    a. ADH.
    b. FSH.
    c. LH.
    d. HRT.
    e. PSA.

51. When protein passes through the nephron, instead of reabsorbing into the blood, it will result in:

    a. hematuria.
    b. albuminuria.
    c. pyuria.
    d. anuria.
    e. polyuria.

52. What is the condition of nonmalignant prostate enlargement?

    a. Erectile dysfunction
    b. Orchitis
    c. Benign prostatic hyperplasia
    d. Cryptorchidism
    e. Epididymitis

53. The laboratory test that increases indicating there is cancer in the prostate gland is:

    a. HPV.
    b. PID.
    c. BPH.
    d. HRT.
    e. PSA.

54. What occurs during the third stage of labor?

    a. There are regular uterine contractions causing the cervix to thin.
    b. The amniotic sac of fluid ruptures.
    c. The cervix completely dilates.
    d. The placenta is delivered.
    e. The baby is delivered through the birth canal.

55. What percent of normal urine is water?

    a. 40%
    b. 50%
    c. 60%
    d. 75%
    e. 95%

56. What medical term means inflammation of the breast?

    a. Mammogram
    b. Mastectomy
    c. Mastitis
    d. Gynecomastia
    e. Mastorrhea

57. Which of these determines the initial health and condition of a newborn?

    a. Apgar score
    b. Birth score
    c. Gestational score
    d. Spontaneous score
    e. Obstetrical score

58. Which of these statements describes characteristics of fraternal twins?

    a. There is a single placenta shared by the two.
    b. They are always the same sex.
    c. They develop from a single egg but two sperm.
    d. There are two eggs and two sperm involved.
    e. They each have an amniotic sac but share a placenta.

59. The substance that is an indicator for pregnancy tests is:

    a. HRT.
    b. HCG.
    c. EDC.
    d. PSA.
    e. FSH.

60. Surgical sterilization in the female involves ligation of the:

    a. uterus.
    b. ovary.
    c. fallopian tube.
    d. follicle.
    e. endometrium.

61. HPV causes:

    a. vaginitis.
    b. chlamydia.
    c. syphilis.
    d. gonorrhea.
    e. genital warts.

62. Menorrhagia is a term that means:

    a. vaginal discharge.
    b. infection of the fallopian tubes.
    c. surgical removal of the uterus.
    d. excessive uterine bleeding.
    e. painful menstruation.

63. The release of an egg from a follicle is:

    a. ovulation.
    b. fertilization.
    c. menstruation.
    d. preovulation.
    e. postmenopausal.

64. An excess of nitrogen waste substances in the blood causes:

    a. hematuria.
    b. uremia.
    c. anemia.
    d. polyuria.
    e. cystitis.

65. The bacteria frequently contaminating urine is:

    a. *Streptococcus*.
    b. gonorrhea.
    c. *E. coli*.
    d. syphilis.
    e. *Staphylococcus*.

66. The presence of numerous white cells and pus in the urine is:

    a. hematuria.
    b. albuminuria.
    c. ketonuria.
    d. glycosuria.
    e. pyuria.

BRIEF EXPLANATIONS

67. Explain the purpose of the placenta and the umbilical cord during pregnancy.

    _____

    _____

    _____

    _____

68. Explain the difference between an abortion, spontaneous abortion, and an induced abortion.

    _____

    _____

    _____

    _____

69. Explain the function of each of these structures of the urinary system.

a. Nephron - _____

b. Renal pelvis - _____

c. Ureter - _____

d. Bladder - _____

e. Urethra - _____

WHAT DO YOU DO?

70. Read the following scenario and respond to the questions with a short answer.

Ms. Peterson just delivered a baby boy and brought the baby for his first check up with the pediatrician. She does not understand why it is important to try to breast feed the baby as opposed to using a bottle and formula. She tells you that she did not understand what the doctor was explaining to her about the benefits of nursing a baby.

a. Write a narrative explanation you could use to help the patient understand the reasons why breast-feeding is beneficial for newborns.

_____

_____

_____

_____

PATIENT EDUCATION

71. The physician asks you to develop an information sheet for female patients explaining why they are more prone to develop UTIs. What information should be included that explains how a UTI begins?

_____

_____

_____

_____

INTERNET RESEARCH

Visit the National Institutes for Health Web site at www.nih.gov, and research the condition of infertility in females. Provide information about the possible causes and types of treatment that will help a woman to become pregnant.

_____

_____

_____

_____

_____

_____

_____

Section III

Administrative Medical Assistant Skills

Chapter Objectives

- Relate the basics of appointment scheduling and management.
- Describe the systems used for scheduling appointments.
- Identify the factors that affect appointment scheduling.
- Follow a set of steps to schedule new patients and return visits.
- Specify three ways to remind patients of appointments.
- Explain how to triage patient emergencies, acutely ill patients, and walk-ins.
- Understand how to handle late patients, delays, cancellations, and missed appointments.
- Schedule inpatient and outpatient admissions and procedures.
- Make referral and consultation appointments with other physicians.
- Follow third-party guidelines to schedule tests and other procedures.
- Schedule hospital admissions for patients.

CAAHEP & ABHES Competencies

CAAHEP

- Discuss pros and cons of various types of appointment management systems.
- Describe scheduling guidelines.
- Recognize office policies and protocols for handling appointments.
- Identify critical information required for scheduling patient admissions and/or procedures.
- Manage appointment schedule, using established priorities.
- Schedule patient admissions and/or procedures.

ABHES

- Apply scheduling principles.
- Scheduling of in- and outpatient procedures.
- Understand procedures for hospital admission and procedures.

TERMINOLOGY MATCHING

Directions: Match the terms in Column A with the definitions in Column B.

Column A

1. _____ Acute
2. _____ Chronic

3. _____ Clustering
4. _____ Constellation of symptoms
5. _____ Consultation
6. _____ Double-booking

7. _____ Fixed scheduling
8. _____ Itinerary
9. _____ Matrix
10. _____ Modified wave

11. _____ Precertification
12. _____ Preferred provider

13. _____ Referral
14. _____ Streaming

15. _____ Third-party payers

16. _____ Wave

Column B

a. The practice of grouping patients with similar problems or needs
b. Scheduling several patients within the same block of time however modifying the types of appointments within the block
c. Scheduling several patients for the same block of time
d. Scheduling of two patients in the same time slot with the same physician
e. Sudden onset of symptoms
f. The patient's care and treatment is actually transferred to the other physician
g. Detailed plan of a trip
h. Long-standing symptoms
i. The insurer must approve the appointment/test in advance
j. The physician wants another physician's opinion about the patient
k. Patients are attached or stuck into one appointment slot
l. Insurance companies, HMOs, and other health care plans that pay patients' medical bills
m. Symptoms occurring together that can signal a specific problem
n. Blocking out the times providers are not available for appointments
o. Assigning appointment lengths based on patients' needs/reason for visit
p. Physicians, hospitals, and others that are in the plan's approved network of providers

DEFINING ABBREVIATIONS

Directions: Provide the specific meaning of each of the following abbreviations. Watch your spelling.

17. CPE: _____

_____

18. EMS: _____

_____

19. ER: _____

_____

20. NPT (NP): _____

_____

21. OV: _____

_____

22. STAT: _____

_____

MAKING IT RIGHT

Each of the following statements is false. Rewrite the statement to make it a true statement.

23. Dr. Smith sent his patient Jamie to Dr. Kline for a consultation. This means care of the patient has been transferred to Dr. Kline.

_____

_____

_____

_____

24. When a parent pays for the health care expense of their child, they are a third-party payer.

_____

_____

_____

_____

25. Precertifications are always completed after the patient received the service. This will ensure an accurate diagnosis is used.

_____

_____

_____

_____

26. You should never ask a patient why they need to be seen. All appointments are scheduled for the same amount of time.

_____

_____

_____

_____

27. You can schedule appointments any time the office is open as the physician will always be available.

_____

_____

_____

_____

MULTIPLE CHOICE

Directions: Choose the best answer for each question.

28. The process of recording the physician's unavailable time on the schedule is known as creating a:

    a. calendar.
    b. itinerary.
    c. matrix.
    d. metric.
    e. preauth.

29. A patient calling with an acute symptom should be scheduled:

    a. in 3 months.
    b. 4 to 6 weeks from the day they call.
    c. not at all, they should go to urgent care.
    d. with a specialist.
    e. as soon as possible.

30. Which of the following represents a system where each hour is broken into equal sections and patients are assigned a set time for their appointment?

    a. Fixed scheduling
    b. Streaming
    c. Wave
    d. Modified wave
    e. Clustering

31. Setting an appointment based on the reason the patient is being seen is known as:

    a. fixed scheduling.
    b. streaming.
    c. wave.
    d. modified wave.
    e. clustering.

32. How much time would you typically allow for a CPE?

    a. 15 minutes
    b. 60 minutes
    c. 5 minutes
    d. 30 minutes
    e. 20 minutes

33. When two patients are scheduled for the exact same time, this is called:

    a. streaming.
    b. matrix.
    c. clustering.
    d. double-booking.
    e. constellation.

34. When you have all of your patients report at 11 AM, for the 11-noon time frame, you are using the _____ scheduling system.

    a. Fixed
    b. Streaming
    c. Wave
    d. Clustering
    e. Modified wave

35. If you were to schedule one major appointment in the first half of an hour and then schedule for brief appointments for the second half of the hour, you would be using which system?

    a. Fixed
    b. Streaming
    c. Wave
    d. Clustering
    e. Modified wave

36. Your office is scheduling all flu vaccines on Tuesdays. What type of scheduling is this?

    a. Fixed
    b. Streaming
    c. Wave
    d. Clustering
    e. Modified wave

37. When a patient is in the office and schedules a return visit, you should:

    a. call them with the information after they get home.
    b. have them call the office when they get home for the information.
    c. provide them with an appointment card.
    d. send all the information by mail.
    e. send the patient a Google appointment reminder.

38. Which of following should be included on a reminder card?

    a. Patient's name, date, and time of appointment
    b. Patient's name, address and phone number, and time of appointment
    c. Physician name, address and phone number, and date of appointment
    d. Patient's name, day, date, and time of appointment, physician's name and phone number
    e. Patient's name, address, and phone number, day, date, and time of appointment

39. Confirmation calls a day or two prior to the patient's appointment greatly reduce the amount of:

    a. complaints.
    b. missed appointments.
    c. cancellations.
    d. rescheduling.
    e. liability.

40. A patient complaining of _____ should be transferred to a nurse or physician due to the nature of the call.

    a. Severe chest pain
    b. Right leg pain
    c. Abdominal discomfort
    d. Low back pain
    e. Nausea and vomiting

41. Which of the following symptoms would require a same-day office appointment?

    a. Chronic low back pain
    b. Follow-up for hypertension
    c. Annual breast exam and pap
    d. Pediatric immunization
    e. Severe vomiting for more than 2 days

42. When certain symptoms appear together, they can signal a specific problem; this is called:

    a. clustering of symptoms.
    b. constellation of symptoms.
    c. review of systems.
    d. consultation of symptoms.
    e. review of symptoms.

43. If a patient does not show for an appointment, you should:

    a. call the patient to see why they missed and ensure they are okay.
    b. cancel the appointment so no one holds it against them.
    c. immediately send the patient a bill.
    d. refuse to allow them to reschedule.
    e. charge them for the missed appointment and reschedule the appointment for 3 months out.

44. Which of the following represents a way to manage a chronically late patient?

    a. Discharge the patient from the physician's care.
    b. Schedule the patient as the first patient of the day.
    c. Schedule the patient at the end of the day.
    d. Refuse to reschedule the patient.
    e. Schedule the patient in the middle of the day.

45. When a patient cancels an appointment, it is important to notate:

    a. who canceled the appointment.
    b. the date the appointment was rescheduled to.
    c. who you schedule in the patient's time slot.
    d. the reason the appointment was canceled.
    e. the time the patient called to cancel.

46. Which of the following procedures should you follow if your physician has to cancel appointments for 3 weeks from today?

    a. First, mail letters and then call any patients still on the schedule the day before the appointment.
    b. First, call patients to reschedule and then send letters to those you can't reach following up with any appointments remaining after 3 to 5 days.
    c. Mail letters informing patients of the cancellation and asking them to call to reschedule with no actions to be taken.
    d. Call the patients and notify them of the need to cancel and reschedule. If they fail to call back, it's their fault.
    e. Reschedule all the appointments to the same time on a different day and mail letter to the patients advising them of the change.

47. When selecting a provider of service for your patients, it is beneficial to the patient if they are:

    a. approved providers.
    b. preferred providers.
    c. primary care providers.
    d. exclusive provider organizations.
    e. nonparticipating providers.

48. When a physician sends a patient to another provider for the sole purpose of obtaining another opinion, it is called a:

    a. third-party payer.
    b. referral.
    c. consultation.
    d. preauthorized visit.
    e. surgical opinion.

49. An itinerary should include which of the following?

    a. Flight information (airline, flight number, seat number, departure date and time, arrival date and time) for both directions
    b. Hotel name, address and phone number, dates of reservations, and reservation number
    c. Ground transportation, car rental or shuttle name, phone number, and reservation number
    d. Meeting or conference information (name, location address and phone number, room number, and registration confirmation number)
    e. All of the above

50. How many copies of the itinerary should be made?

    a. 3
    b. 4
    c. 2
    d. 1
    e. 5

51. Copies of the itinerary should be given to the:

    a. hospital, physician, and the office.
    b. physician, physician's family, and the hospital.
    c. emergency room, office, and the hospital.
    d. physician, physician's family, and the office.
    e. hospital, physician, and the patients.

52. Once a patient is scheduled for a consultation with another provider, your office should send:

    a. copies of complete medical records and consultation request.
    b. consultation request form and precertification.
    c. copies of pertinent medical records, consultation form, and precertification.
    d. copies of complete medical records.
    e. consultation form and precertification.

BRIEF EXPLANATIONS

53. Explain why it is important to know the reason for a patient's visit.

    _____

    _____

    _____

    _____

54. Describe tasks the physician may need time to complete outside of seeing patients.

    _____

    _____

    _____

    _____

55. List three questions you would want to ask a patient calling to schedule an appointment.

_____

_____

_____

_____

56. Describe two systems of scheduling that can be used in the medical office.

_____

_____

_____

_____

57. Using the two systems above, list two positives and two negatives for each system.

_____

_____

_____

_____

58. List three things to consider when determining the amount of time an appointment will require.

_____

_____

_____

_____

WHAT DO YOU DO?

59. Read the following scenario and respond to the questions with a short answer.

    You scheduled a patient for an MRI 2 weeks ago at an outside facility. You completed the precertification request online and it was pending. The patient called the facility and changed the MRI to an earlier date without notifying you. Today, you learned that the insurance denied the MRI. When you call the patient, he explains he already completed the MRI and is very upset.

    a. What is your immediate response to this situation?

    _____

    _____

    _____

    _____

    b. Is there anything that you or the physician can do about the MRI being denied?

    _____

    _____

    _____

c. If the physician completes a peer-to-peer and it is determined that the MRI will still not be covered, who will be responsible for the bill?

_____

_____

_____

_____

d. What steps can you take to prevent this from happening again with other patients?

_____

_____

_____

_____

PATIENT EDUCATION

60. Write a short narrative script that you can use to provide patient education explaining the importance of preauthorization/precertification of certain procedures. Detail protocol that would be beneficial to both you and the patient.

_____

_____

_____

_____

INTERNET RESEARCH

Visit the Aetna insurance precertification Web site at https://www.aetna.com/health-care-professionals/precertification.html. Click on "check our precertification lists" and then "search by code." Enter the following CPT codes 72146, 72147, 72148, and 70336. Which of the codes require precertification? List the contact number you would call to precertify these procedures in your area.

_____

_____

_____

_____

_____

_____

_____

Procedure 10-1 | Making Appointments for New Patients

Name: _____ Date: _____ Time: _____ Grade: _____

Equipment: Appointment book (manual or electronic); patient information

Performance Requirement: Student will perform this skill with ____% accuracy not to exceed _____ minutes. (Instructor will determine the point value for each step, % accuracy, and minutes required.)

Performance Checklist

Point Value	Performance Points Earned	Procedure Steps
		1. Obtain the patient's full name, address, day and evening phone numbers, reason for the visit, and name of who referred the patient.
		2. Explain the office's payment policy. Ask the patient to bring insurance information to the office. You should also verify insurance to determine whether your office participates in their plan.
		3. Make sure the patient knows where the office is located. Give directions if needed.
		4. Ask the patient if it's acceptable to call them at home or work.
		5. Double-check your appointment book or computer screen to make sure you have recorded the appointment for the correct date and time.
		6. Before hanging up, confirm the day, date, and time of the appointment with the patient.
		7. If another physician referred the patient, make a note to contact the referring physician's office for copies of the patient's records.

CALCULATION

Total Points Possible: _____

Total Points Earned: _____

Points Earned/Points Possible = _____%

Student completion time (minutes): _____

PASS   FAIL   COMMENTS:

_____

Student's signature _____ Date _____

Instructor's signature _____ Date _____

Procedure 10-2	Making Appointments for Established Patients

Name: _____ Date: _____ Time: _____ Grade: _____

Equipment: Appointment book (manual or electronic) and patient information

Performance Requirement: Student will perform this skill with ____% accuracy not to exceed _____ minutes. (Instructor will determine the point value for each step, % accuracy, and minutes required.)

Performance Checklist

Point Value	Performance Points Earned	Procedure Steps
		1. Find out the reason for the return visit. If a specific test is to be done, check the schedule to see when the equipment is available.
		2. Offer the patient a specific date and time. If the patient doesn't agree, offer one or two other dates and times.
		3. Enter the patient's name and telephone contact number in the appointment book or the computer. Also, confirm their current insurance to verify that they are still with a participating plan.
		4. Place the information on an appointment card and give it to the patient. Repeat aloud to the patient the day, date, and time of the appointment as you hand over the card.
		5. Double-check your record of the appointment to be sure you have not made an error.
		6. End your conversation with a pleasant word and smile.

CALCULATION

Total Points Possible: _____

Total Points Earned: _____

Points Earned/Points Possible = _____%

Student completion time (minutes): _____

PASS   FAIL   COMMENTS:

_____

Student's signature _____ Date _____

Instructor's signature _____ Date _____

Procedure 10-3 Making Appointments for Patients in Other Facilities

Name: _____ Date: _____ Time: _____ Grade: _____

Equipment: Patient information including insurance, name of test or appointment needed, patient diagnosis, reason for test or appointment, name of physician ordering, physician's NPI or tax ID number, and patient's record (EHR).

Performance Requirement: Student will perform this skill with ____% accuracy not to exceed _____ minutes. (Instructor will determine the point value for each step, % accuracy, and minutes required.)

Performance Checklist

Point Value	Performance Points Earned	Procedure Steps
		1. Make certain that the requirements of the patient's health care plan are met.
		2. Refer to the preferred provider list for the patient's health care plan and call a provider on this list.
		3. Have the following information available when you call the provider: • The name and phone number of your office and physician • The patient's name, address, and phone number • The reason the patient is being sent to the other provider • How urgent it is that the patient be seen • The approval number from the patient's health care plan if precertification is required
		4. Record the date and time of the call as well as the name of the person you spoke with.
		5. Ask the person you're calling to notify you if the patient doesn't keep the appointment.
		6. Document the name, address, and phone number of the place you are sending the patient and the date and time of the patient's appointment. Record information on an appointment card or stationary and give or mail to patient.

CALCULATION

Total Points Possible: _____

Total Points Earned: _____

Points Earned/Points Possible = _____%

Student completion time (minutes): _____

PASS   FAIL   COMMENTS:

_____

Student's signature _____ Date _____

Instructor's signature _____ Date _____

11 Medical Documentation

Chapter Objectives

- List information contained in a medical record.
- Establish and maintain the medical record.
- Contrast the ways in which medical records can be organized.
- Discuss security of medical records.
- Explain how to make entries in a patient's medical record.
- Describe how to make corrections in medical records.
- Document appropriately.
- Explain proper access and use of medical records.

CAAHEP & ABHES Competencies

CAAHEP

- Define types of information contained in the patient's medical record.
- Identify methods of organizing the patient's medical record.
- Identify equipment and supplies needed to create, maintain, and store medical records.
- Describe filing indexing rules.
- Differentiate between electronic medical records (EMR) and a practice management system.
- Create a patient's medical record.
- Organize a patient's medical record.
- File patient medical records.
- Utilize an EMR.
- Input patient data utilizing a practice management system.
- Explain the importance of data backup.
- Explain meaningful use as it applies to EMR.

ABHES

- Utilize electronic medical records (EMR) and practice management systems.
- Comply with federal, state, and local laws relating to exchange of information.
- Describe elements of meaningful use and reports generated.
- Demonstrate understanding of records management.

TERMINOLOGY MATCHING

Directions: Match the terms in Column A with the definitions in Column B.

Column A

1. _____ Active records
2. _____ Assessment
3. _____ Closed records
4. _____ Consultation reports
5. _____ Database
6. _____ Flow sheet
7. _____ Inactive records
8. _____ Narrative style
9. _____ Numeric filing systems
10. _____ Objective
11. _____ Progress note
12. _____ Radiographic reports
13. _____ Secondary records
14. _____ Subject filing
15. _____ Subjective
16. _____ Worker's compensation

Column B

a. Reports from other physicians with whom the patient's physician asked to consult about the patient
b. Assign a six-digit number to each patient
c. Records of patients who have not been seen in 3 or more years
d. Reports of x-rays, CT scans, MRIs, and similar studies
e. The records of patients who have been seen recently
f. System in which records are grouped alphabetically according to their subject
g. Health insurance law requires employers to have for workers who suffer job-related injuries
h. Charts of patients who have ended their relationship with the physician
i. Record each contact with a patient
j. A form that allows information to be recorded in a table or on a graph
k. Records received from another physician, hospital, or other source
l. Information the medical assistant and physician observe about the patient
m. Written out as you would speak
n. The diagnosis made by the physician
o. Patient's information including chief complaint and present illness
p. Direct statement or description from the patient telling about his or her own condition

DEFINING ABBREVIATIONS

Directions: Provide the specific meaning of each of the following abbreviations. Watch your spelling.

17. CC: _____

_____

18. EHR: _____

_____

19. FMH: _____

_____

20. HPI: _____

_____

21. POMR: _____

_____

22. PMH: _____

_____

23. ROS: _____

_____

24. SH: _____

_____

25. SOAP: _____

_____

26. SOMR: _____

_____

MAKING IT RIGHT

Each of the following statements is false. Rewrite the statement to make it a true statement.

27. If an individual wished to file a compliancy complaint, they must do so in person. The office has 90 days to investigate and respond. Often, no action is needed.

_____

_____

_____

_____

28. A patient's health record should be maintained in an orderly fashion. All information must be kept in chronological order starting from the first visit and descending to the most recent.

_____

_____

_____

_____

29. The most common method of documenting a patient's visit is the SOAP format. Each letter of SOAP represents a part of the exam/visit. Subjective is anything the physician or medical assistant observes, objective is only information that the patient can give (like level of pain), assessment is physical exam, and plan is the diagnosis.

_____

_____

_____

_____

30. An established patient is injured at work. His employer's Worker's Compensation Insurance contacted the office to arrange an appointment and discuss payment. Despite this being a work-related injury, it is charted in the patient's record along with all his other visits. This way, when they request medical records, they can see everything the patient is being treated for, just in case it affects his recovery.

_____

_____

_____

_____

31. When documenting, the rule is "less is more." You should document the bare minimum; this way, if the chart is called into question during a malpractice case, the physician will be able to explain exactly what happened. This way, this information is clear and concise since the physician will be explaining everything in person.

_____

_____

_____

_____

MULTIPLE CHOICE

Directions: Choose the best answer for each question.

32. Which of the following is the official record of changes in a patient's medical condition?

   a. Insurance claim form
   b. Electronic health record
   c. Research data form
   d. Appointment log
   e. Pain diary

33. Prior to releasing any information from a patient's record, you must have proper authorization from the:

   a. patient's insurance.
   b. physician's attorney.
   c. patient.
   d. patient's attorney.
   e. office manager.

34. In the medical record, the patient demographics would be considered:

   a. personal information.
   b. clinical information.
   c. administrative information.
   d. personal history.
   e. social history.

35. The patient's explanation as to why they came to see the physician, usually expressed in the patient's own words, is referred to the:

   a. history of present illness.
   b. diagnosis.
   c. social history.
   d. past medical history.
   e. chief complaint.

36. When a review of major illnesses of parents and grandparents, aunts and uncles, and brothers and sisters is performed is referred to as:

    a. past medical history.
    b. review of systems.
    c. social history.
    d. family medical history.
    e. history of present illness.

37. The patient's dietary habits as well as drinking, smoking, and drug habits would be listed under which of the following?

    a. Social history
    b. Family medical history
    c. History of present illness
    d. Past medical history
    e. Review of systems

38. Under which heading would you find patient's major illnesses, surgeries, and hospitalizations?

    a. Social history
    b. Family medical history
    c. History of present illness
    d. Past medical history
    e. Review of systems

39. The patient's complaint stated in medical terms, with times and details, would be listed under which of the following headings?

    a. Social history
    b. Family medical history
    c. History of present illness
    d. Past medical history
    e. Review of systems

40. When the physician performs an examination of the body systems to look for problems not yet identified, it is listed under which of the following headings?

    a. Social history
    b. Family medical history
    c. History of present illness
    d. Past medical history
    e. Review of systems

41. Which of following represents the correct meaning for the abbreviation AP?

    a. Appointment
    b. Anteroposterior
    c. Appetite
    d. Approved
    e. Appeal

42. The abbreviation *hs* means:

    a. hours of school.
    b. morning.
    c. afternoon.
    d. hours of sleep.
    e. hours of suffering.

43. Which of the following is the meaning of the abbreviation LLE?

    a. Left leg exam
    b. Left lower eczema
    c. Left lower extremity
    d. Lower lip excision
    e. Left leg eczema

44. The abbreviation *p.c.* means:

    a. post confinement.
    b. after conception.
    c. before conception.
    d. before a meal.
    e. after a meal.

45. The abbreviation *s/p* means:

    a. status post.
    b. surgical prep.
    c. surgical procedure.
    d. schedule procedure.
    e. stat procedure.

46. Phone calls from patients are documented using which of the following styles?

    a. SOAP
    b. POMR
    c. Narrative
    d. SOMR
    e. Focus

47. Which of the following represents good management of an office's electronic medical records?

    a. Back up all files nightly on a thumb drive to take home.
    b. Scan new items in patients' records accurately and in a timely manner.
    c. Enter information on patient care as briefly as possible and as time permits.
    d. New patient charts should be created with no regard for accuracy.
    e. All of the above.

48. Medical records are classified in three categories:

    a. new, established, and stored.
    b. current, noncurrent, and destroyed.
    c. active, closed, and stored.
    d. active, inactive, and closed.
    e. current, inactive, and destroyed.

49. Records of patients who have been seen within the past 3 years are referred to as:

    a. active.
    b. inactive.
    c. closed.
    d. new.
    e. stored.

50. Records of patients who have ended/terminated their care with the physician are referred to as:

    a. active.
    b. inactive.
    c. closed.
    d. new.
    e. stored.

51. Medical records should be kept:

    a. for 5 to 6 years after care has ended.
    b. permanently.
    c. for 60 days after care has ended.
    d. until care is transferred to another physician.
    e. until the patient is deceased.

52. Geographic filing would be used to maintain what type of files?

    a. Patient medical records
    b. Research studies
    c. Inventory
    d. Accounts payable
    e. Accounts receivable

53. Chronological filing systems would be used to maintain:

    a. patient medical records.
    b. research studies.
    c. inventory.
    d. accounts payable.
    e. accounts receivable.

54. The abbreviation *a* means:

    a. before.
    b. after.
    c. with.
    d. without.
    e. always.

55. Which of the following represents the meaning of the abbreviation p?

    a. Before
    b. After
    c. With
    d. Without
    e. Always

56. The abbreviation c means:

    a. before.
    b. after.
    c. with.
    d. without.
    e. constant.

57. The abbreviation s means:

    a. before.
    b. after.
    c. with.
    d. without.
    e. sudden.

58. Which of the following represents the meaning of the abbreviation Hx?

    a. History
    b. Prognosis
    c. Diagnosis
    d. Symptoms
    e. Hysterectomy

59. The abbreviation CPE means:

    a. continue physical exercise.
    b. continue physical education.
    c. complete psychological exam.
    d. current professional education.
    e. complete physical exam.

60. The abbreviation NKDA means:

    a. no potassium dietary aids.
    b. not known; didn't ask.
    c. no known drug allergies.
    d. no known dietary allergies.
    e. no known diabetic acidosis.

BRIEF EXPLANATIONS

61. Laura Smith, a patient of Dr. Jones, is requesting the release of her medical records to another physician. Laura wants your office to release your records and copies of records from her previous physician. Explain how you will handle this situation.

    _____

    _____

    _____

    _____

62. Information within a patient's medical records is confidential and should not be released without the patient's consent. Medical records can be used for other purposes as well. Explain how information gathered from medical records can be used.

    _____

    _____

    _____

    _____

63. Explain how a POMR is organized and why it would be helpful.

_____

_____

_____

_____

64. Describe the function of an SOMR. What are the benefits of this type of record organization?

_____

_____

_____

_____

65. Provide an example of a flow sheet that might be used in a physician office. How is the use of a flow sheet beneficial to patient care.

_____

_____

_____

_____

66. Medical records are legal documents. As a medical assistant, explain actions you can take to ensure that they represent your office well?

_____

_____

_____

_____

WHAT DO YOU DO?

67. It's an extremely busy day at the office. You feel rushed and overwhelmed but you just keep moving on. The patient you are discharging asked the physician to write a script for their medication as they wanted to change pharmacies and didn't have the information with them. As you are discharging the patient, he says he has changed his mind about his pharmacy and asks if you can just send the order over electronically to the pharmacy on file so it will be ready when he gets there. You rush to the computer to enter the order before moving on to the next patient. In your rush, you misread the order lisinopril 2.5 mg as lisinopril 12.5 mg.

    a. What steps could have been taken to avoid this error?

    _____

    _____

    _____

    _____

b. The pharmacy calls to confirm the order as it represents a much higher dose than usual. You are in a room with a patient and the physician notes have not yet been transcribed so the medical assistant taking the call confirmed your order for 12.5 mg without noting it in the patient chart. What steps should have been taken in this case?

_____

_____

_____

_____

c. Two days later, the ER calls as the patient arrived via ambulance after losing consciousness at the mall. Patient presents with severe hypotension. The physician speaks with the ER to confirm medications and discovers the medication error. Could malpractice be proven in this case?

_____

_____

_____

_____

d. What steps should be followed to avoid such errors in the office?

_____

_____

_____

_____

PATIENT EDUCATION

68. Write a short narrative outlining how you would explain secondary release of medical records to a patient.

_____

_____

_____

_____

INTERNET RESEARCH

In this chapter, we learned that medical documentation is vital to quality patient care. Proper documentation also protects the physician(s) against wrongful lawsuits and claims of medical billing fraud. Use the www.cms.gov Web site and search "errors in medical documentation." Select one of the documents to review and provide a brief summary of the article.

_____

_____

_____

_____

_____

12 Medical Insurance Coding

Chapter Objectives

- Explain what coding is and why it is used.
- Describe the relationship between diagnostic coding, procedural coding, and reimbursement.
- Describe how the ICD-10-CM is organized.
- List the steps in identifying a proper diagnostic code.
- Name the common errors in diagnostic coding.
- Perform diagnostic coding.
- Describe how the CPT-4 is organized and used.
- Summarize the factors that determine which E/M code to assign a patient visit.
- Understand HCPCS codes and surgical packages.
- Perform procedural coding.
- Demonstrate understanding of upcoding and downcoding.
- Determine medical necessity as it applies to coding.
- Understand the importance of communication with medical providers to ensure accurate code selection.

CAAHEP & ABHES Competencies

CAAHEP

- Describe how to use the most current procedural coding system.
- Describe how to use the most current diagnostic coding classification system.
- Describe how to use the most current HCPCS level II coding system.
- Discuss the effects of upcoding and downcoding.
- Define medical necessity as it applies to procedural and diagnostic coding.
- Perform procedural coding.
- Perform diagnostic coding.
- Utilize medical necessity guidelines.
- Utilize tactful communication skills with medical providers to ensure accurate code selection.

ABHES

- Perform diagnostic and procedural coding.

TERMINOLOGY MATCHING

Directions: Match the terms in Column A with the definitions in Column B.

Column A

1. _____ Alphanumeric
2. _____ Bundled
3. _____ Comorbidity
4. _____ Diagnostic codes
5. _____ Downcoding
6. _____ Etiology
7. _____ Global surgical follow-up
8. _____ Initial encounter

9. _____ Key components

10. _____ Late effects
11. _____ Medical necessity
12. _____ Modifiers

13. _____ Physical status modifier

14. _____ Procedure codes
15. _____ Primary diagnosis

16. _____ Subsequent encounter

17. _____ Sequela
18. _____ Unbundled
19. _____ Upcoding

Column B

a. More than one disease or condition occurring at the same time
b. The first time seeing the patient
c. Added to a code as they offer additional special information
d. Coding for less than the actual service provided
e. Codes that describe services provided to the patient
f. The use of numbers and letters to create a code
g. The cause of the disease
h. Code for the diagnosis, complaint, or reason the patient sought attention that day
i. An action of separating codes out of a bundled package as a means of charging more
j. History, physical examination, and medical decision making
k. Submitting a code for a service the physician hasn't performed
l. The procedure or service billed was reasonable for the patient's medical condition
m. The codes from all the tests/procedures performed together are combined into one code
n. Another name for subsequent encounter
o. An inclusive package of all the procedures and visits surrounding a surgical procedure
p. Tells the patient's condition, at the time of anesthesia administration
q. Codes are used to identify the reason the patient is seeking care
r. Indicates follow-up encounters
s. Conditions that result from a past injury or illness

DEFINING ABBREVIATIONS

Directions: Provide the specific meaning of each of the following abbreviations. Watch your spelling.

20. CMS: _____

_____

21. CPT-4: _____

_____

22. E/M: _____

_____

23. HCPCS: _____

_____

24. HIPAA: _____

_____

25. ICD-10-CM: _____

_____

26. NCHS: _____

_____

27. OIG: _____

_____

28. WHO: _____

_____

MAKING IT RIGHT

Each of the following statements is false. Rewrite the statement to make it a true statement.

29. Downcoding is an unethical and illegal practice where a code less than the service provided is used. Upcoding is an ethical practice of using a code greater than the service provided as a means of increasing practice earnings.

_____

_____

_____

_____

30. Diagnostic codes are found in the CPT-4, and procedural codes are located in the ICD-10-CM. These codes ensure proper reimbursement of services.

_____

_____

_____

_____

31. When the physician records a diagnosis of "rule out," you should assume the patient has that condition and code accordingly.

_____

_____

_____

_____

32. Codes for supplies and services, such as bandages or ambulance, can be found in the CPT-4 book.

_____

_____

_____

_____

33. When coding multiple diagnoses on a patient, the order in which appear is irrelevant.

_____

_____

_____

_____

MULTIPLE CHOICE

Directions: Choose the best answer for each question.

34. A chest x-ray is performed on a patient with a diagnosis of otitis media (ear infection). The insurance denies the claim stating that the diagnosis does not support the procedure based on:

    a. deductible.
    b. medical necessity.
    c. coinsurance.
    d. comorbidity.
    e. downcoding.

35. Diagnostic codes can be found in which of the following books?

    a. ICD-10-CM
    b. CPT
    c. HCPCS
    d. WHO
    e. CMS

36. Which of the following books would be used to code procedures?

    a. CMS
    b. HCPCS
    c. CPT
    d. ICD-10-CM
    e. WHO

37. Which of the following books would contain codes not listed in the CPT book?
    a. CMS
    b. CPT
    c. ICD-10-CM
    d. WHO
    e. HCPCS

38. When a procedure code for services greater than those provided is used, this is called:

    a. downcoding.
    b. coding.
    c. upcycling.
    d. upcoding.
    e. downcycling.

39. If a physician uses a code for services less than those provided, it would result in a/an:

    a. investigation.
    b. overpayment.
    c. underpayment.
    d. upcode.
    e. legal action.

40. A red dot at the margin of an ICD-10-CM code means:

    a. stop and check for additional digits.
    b. code the underlying cause first.
    c. use this code for a newborn only.
    d. two codes are likely needed to fully explain the condition.
    e. this code has been deleted.

41. ICD-10-CM codes that begin with letters V to Y are used to code which of the following?

    a. Immunizations
    b. Well-care examinations
    c. External causes
    d. Pregnancy
    e. Use of an AED

42. ICD-10-CM codes that begin with Z are used to code:

    a. problems arising from external causes.
    b. annual well-care examinations.
    c. emergency situations requiring an AED.
    d. accidental poisoning.
    e. issues occurring from therapeutic use of a medication.

43. ICD-10 codes can be up to _____ characters in length.

    a. 4
    b. 5
    c. 6
    d. 7
    e. 8

44. In diagnostic coding, there will be times when a space doesn't require a digit. In such incidents, a placeholder is needed. Which letter below represents an ICD-10 placeholder?

    a. Z
    b. V
    c. X
    d. A
    e. B

45. Conditions that are a result of past injury or illness are called _____. They are present long after treatment of the injury or illness.

    a. terminal.
    b. long term.
    c. systemic.
    d. after effects.
    e. late effects.

46. If a patient presents with medical concerns following a drug interaction caused by someone's deliberate attempt to cause harm to code, you would first locate the drug and then which of the following circumstances?

    a. Accidental poisoning
    b. Therapeutic use
    c. Suicide attempt
    d. Assault
    e. Undetermined

47. If a patient has a diagnosis of acute upper respiratory infection, what is the main term?

    a. Acute
    b. Upper
    c. Respiratory
    d. Infection
    e. URI

48. If a patient is seen in the office for gastroenteritis and also has a diagnosis of diabetes mellitus type I, morbid obesity, hypertension, and hypothyroidism. Which diagnosis should be used as the primary diagnosis?

    a. Gastroenteritis
    b. Diabetes mellitus type I
    c. Morbid obesity
    d. Hypertension
    e. Hypothyroidism

49. In cases, such as the one in question 48, where the patient has multiple diseases or conditions occurring at the same time, it is referred to as:

    a. multiple diagnoses.
    b. codiagnoses.
    c. comorbidity.
    d. late effects.
    e. upcoding.

50. A patient reports to the office with the CC of severe headaches × 2 weeks and one episode of loss of consciousness lasting about 2 minutes. The physician orders an MRI and records a diagnosis of rule out brain tumor. What will you code as the diagnosis/diagnoses for today's visit?

    a. Brain tumor and severe headache
    b. Rule out brain tumor and loss of consciousness (approximately 2 minutes)
    c. Severe headache and loss of consciousness (approximately 2 minutes)
    d. Brain tumor with loss of consciousness (approximately 2 minutes)
    e. Rule out brain tumor and severe headache

51. CPT codes are used to code procedures and consist of:

    a. five characters both letters and numbers.
    b. seven alphanumeric characters.
    c. five letters.
    d. seven numbers.
    e. five numbers.

52. Routine office visit codes are located in which of the following sections of the CPT?

    a. Medicine
    b. Evaluation and Management
    c. Pathology and Laboratory
    d. Radiology
    e. Surgery

53. A _____ can be added to a CPT code to provide additional, special information about the service.

    a. asterisk
    b. status
    c. appendix
    d. modifier
    e. sequela

54. This symbol ►◄ in the CPT book indicates:

    a. new or revised text.
    b. a new code.
    c. a revised code.
    d. an add-on code.
    e. the code is modifier –51 exempt.

55. In the CPT book, the symbol □ indicates:

    a. a revised code.
    b. resequenced codes.
    c. the code is modifier –51 exempt.
    d. a recycled or reinstated code.
    e. an add-on code.

56. Codes for medication would be found in which of the following coding books?

    a. ICD-10-CM
    b. CPT-4
    c. WHO
    d. CMS
    e. HCPCS

57. Which of following represents a special modifier that identifies a patient's condition at the time of anesthesia?

    a. Apgar modifier
    b. Physical status modifier
    c. –51
    d. –25
    e. Sedation modifier

58. The three key components used in determining an E/M code include which of the following?

    a. Coordination of care, time, and counseling
    b. Nature of presenting problem, medical decision making, and physical examination
    c. History, nature of presenting problem, and time
    d. History, physical examination, and medical decision making
    e. Time, counseling, and nature of presenting problem

BRIEF EXPLANATIONS

59. Describe the process of coding a neoplasm, and include all information that would be needed to properly code.

    _____

    _____

    _____

    _____

60. Explain the purpose and use of the three volumes within the ICD-10-CM.

_____

_____

_____

_____

61. Summarize the five circumstances used to code harm caused from a drug or other substance.

_____

_____

_____

_____

62. Explain the three key components used in determining the level of service for E/M codes.

_____

_____

_____

_____

63. List the seven factors used to determine the proper E/M code.

_____

_____

_____

_____

64. Describe the purpose of each of the appendices listed in the CPT-4 book.

_____

_____

_____

_____

WHAT DO YOU DO?

65. Read the following scenario and respond to the questions with a short answer.

John Jacobs, a new patient, was seen today for exercise-induced chest pain. John has an extensive PMH including open heart surgery 3 years ago. His primary care physician retired, and his cardiologist has moved to another state. John has a lengthy FH. Dr. Jones spent 75 minutes face to face with the patient. He ordered an ECG, performed in the office, along with thallium cardiac stress test to be performed at the hospital this afternoon. Dr. Jones has also ordered stat labs, also to be done at the hospital. Dr. Jones noted significant abnormalities on the ECG. He diagnosed the patient with third-degree AV block and hypertension.

a. What procedures will you bill for? What level of service will you use for the office visit?

_____

_____

_____

b. Is a modifier necessary for any of the services performed today?

_____

_____

_____

_____

c. What diagnosis or diagnoses will you code?

_____

_____

_____

_____

d. Which diagnosis is primary?

_____

_____

_____

_____

PATIENT EDUCATION

66. Write a short narrative script that you can use to explain the process of assigning evaluation and management (E/M) procedure codes. This information will be helpful when assisting others, including the physician, with selecting proper codes.

_____

_____

_____

_____

INTERNET RESEARCH

Visit the Center for Medicare and Medicaid Services Web site at www.cms.gov, and search for "provider resources." Select a current resource to review (article or video). Give a brief summary of information you gained from this resource.

_____

_____

_____

_____

_____

_____

_____

Procedure 12-1 | Coding a Diagnosis or Diagnoses

Name: _____ Date: _____ Time: _____ Grade: _____

Equipment: Patient records of diagnosis/diagnoses and treatment and current ICD coding book

Performance Requirement: Student will perform this skill with ____% accuracy not to exceed _____ minutes. (Instructor will determine the point value for each step, % accuracy, and minutes required.)

Performance Checklist

Point Value	Performance Points Earned	Procedure Steps
		1. Using the primary diagnosis, locate the main term (or cause) within the diagnosis.
		2. Locate the main term in the alphabetic section of the ICD coding book procedure.
		3. Refer to the additional descriptive terms or information within the diagnosis.
		4. Follow any special instructions given within the coding book.
		5. Cross-reference the selected code with the numeric section of the ICD coding book. Read through the descriptive of the code selected. Look for any additional digit requirements to ensure your code fully describes the diagnosis.
		6. Assign the code

CALCULATION

Total Points Possible: _____

Total Points Earned: _____

Points Earned/Points Possible = _____%

Student completion time (minutes): _____

PASS   FAIL   COMMENTS:

_____

Student's signature _____ Date _____

Instructor's signature_____ Date _____

Procedure 12-2 Assigning a Procedural Code

Name: _____ Date: _____ Time: _____ Grade: _____

Equipment: Patient chart, billing sheet with procedures selected, and current edition of CPT-4

Performance Requirement: Student will perform this skill with _____% accuracy not to exceed _____ minutes. (Instructor will determine the point value for each step, % accuracy, and minutes required.)

Performance Checklist

Point Value	Performance Points Earned	Procedure Steps
		1. Identify the exact service or procedure performed.
		2. Using the index in the book of the CPT book, locate the procedure. Utilize the code or code range to cross-reference to the front of the book. *Important note: Even if only one code is listed for a particular service, it must be cross-referenced to ensure that it is the correct code.*
		3. Locate the code or code range and read through the primary procedure(s) listed. Select the primary procedure that describes the service or procedure performed.
		4. Read through the indented description below the code you selected. Locate the code that matches the procedure in as much detail as possible.
		5. Be sure to read through the "Special Guidelines" section located at the front of the coding section to ensure that all guidelines are followed.
		6. Determine if a modifier is needed. Remember, any unusual or special circumstance will require a modifier.
		7. If a modifier is needed, or if you are uncertain, review the modifier summaries on the front cover to locate possible modifiers. Then, cross-reference selected modifiers to the Modifier Appendix. Review the details of each modifier to select the correct one.
		8. Assign the selected code with modifier(s), if required.

(Continued)

Procedure 12-2   Assigning a Procedural Code (*Continued*)

CALCULATION

Total Points Possible: _____

Total Points Earned: _____

Points Earned/Points Possible = _____%

Student completion time (minutes): _____

PASS   FAIL   COMMENTS:

_____

Student's signature _____   Date _____

Instructor's signature _____   Date _____

13 Managing Medical Office Finances

Chapter Objectives

- Explain fee schedules and describe the main forms of payment.
- Summarize the process of identifying and collecting unpaid bills.
- Perform billing and collection procedures.
- Charge and payment entry.
- Perform accounts receivable procedures.
- Post adjustments.
- Process credit balance.
- Post NSF checks.
- Post collection agency payments.
- Process refunds.
- Describe how medical offices use bank services.
- Prepare a bank deposit.
- Identify accounts payable functions and relate how they are handled.

CAAHEP & ABHES Competencies

CAAHEP

- Define common bookkeeping terms.
- Describe banking procedures commonly used in the medical office.
- Identify precautions for accepting common types of payments.
- Describe types of adjustments made to patient accounts.
- Identify types of information required for patient billing.
- Explain patient financial obligations for office services.
- Perform accounts receivable procedures (posting of charges, payments, and adjustments).
- Prepare a bank deposit.
- Obtain accurate patient billing information.
- Demonstrate professionalism when discussing patient's financial obligations.

ABHES

- Demonstrate proper medical office billing and collection procedures.
- Explain accounts payable and accounts receivable.
- Demonstrate ability to post charges, payments, and adjustments.
- Explain payment procedures for credit balance, nonsufficient funds, and refunds.

TERMINOLOGY MATCHING

Directions: Match the terms in Column A with the definitions in Column B.

Column A

1. _____ Accounting
2. _____ Accounts payable
3. _____ Accounts receivable
4. _____ Adjustments
5. _____ Aging schedule
6. _____ Bookkeeping
7. _____ Charges
8. _____ Coinsurance
9. _____ Collections
10. _____ Co-payment
11. _____ Credit
12. _____ Credit balance
13. _____ Cycle billing
14. _____ Debit
15. _____ Deductible
16. _____ Dunning
17. _____ Extension of credit
18. _____ Fee schedule
19. _____ Nonsufficient funds check
20. _____ Packing slip
21. _____ Posting
22. _____ Restrictive endorsement

Column B

a. Money owed to the office from patient accounts
b. A billing system that divides accounts alphabetically and bills them at separate intervals during the month
c. Amount owed by the insured/patient at time of service
d. The patient doesn't have enough money in his or her account for the bank to pay a check that he or she wrote.
e. Allowing a patient to pay on his or her account balance based on an established contractual agreement.
f. An organized system for keeping track of a business's finances
g. Aging of accounts typically by 30, 60, 90, and 120 or more days past due
h. Means the program saves activity for that day in the system for that month and resets the daily balance for your next day
i. Money the office owes for operating expenses
j. A reduction to what is owed
k. An accounting activity that keeps an organized record of a business's financial activities
l. A subtraction from the amount owed with no monetary exchange
m. An addition to what is owed
n. An overpayment on a patient's account, recorded in brackets
o. Allows you to set parameters with messages to be added onto statements when printing
p. An increase on the accounts receivable balance
q. Lists the items the delivery contains
r. Writing or stamping the name of the physician or medical office, bank name, and account number on the back of the check
s. A list of charges for specific medical procedures
t. Contracted percentage owed by the insured/patient
u. Annual amount owed by the insured prior to insurance payment
v. The process of collecting money to pay on an account.

DEFINING ABBREVIATIONS

Directions: Provide the specific meaning of each of the following abbreviations. Watch your spelling.

23. EOB: _____
_____

24. FICA: _____

_____

25. FIT: _____

_____

26. FUTA: _____

_____

27. IRS: _____

_____

28. NSF: _____

_____

29. RBRVS: _____

_____

30. RVU: _____

_____

31. UCR: _____

_____

32. W-4: _____

_____

MAKING IT RIGHT

Each of the following statements is false. Rewrite the statement to make it a true statement.

33. Adjustments are the same as payments; however, they are only used when the payment is made by credit card.

_____

_____

_____

_____

34. Once you receive the EOB from insurance, you can calculate the amount the patient owes to the office. You do this by totaling the following: deductible owed, coinsurance or co-payment due, and the difference between what was billed and what the insurance allowed.

_____

_____

_____

_____

35. When extending credit to patients, you can choose which patients you want to offer this option to.

_____

_____

_____

_____

36. Cycle billing is when you mail all patient statements once a month on the same date.

_____

_____

_____

_____

37. The Fair Debt Collections Act allows you to do whatever it takes to collection fees owed to your office, including calling patients at work.

_____

_____

_____

_____

MULTIPLE CHOICE

Directions: Choose the best answer for each question.

38. Insurance companies utilize _____ to determine what they will pay for each service.

   a. EOB and UCR
   b. RBRVS and UCR
   c. RVU and the physician's fee schedule
   d. the physician's fee schedule and EOB
   e. RBRVS and FIT

39. A list of charges for each service performed in the office is referred to as a:

   a. FIT.
   b. price sheet.
   c. charge slip.
   d. UCR.
   e. fee schedule.

40. Which of the following represents a good collection practice?

   a. Waiting to collect payments until after insurance has paid
   b. Offering a 20% discount if the patient pays their co-payment within 30 days
   c. Collecting the co-payment at the time of service
   d. Not making a copy of the insurance card
   e. Agreeing to bill the patient's neighbor

41. A subtraction from the amount owed on a patient's account without a monetary exchange is referred to as a/an:

    a. adjustment.
    b. payment.
    c. charge.
    d. debit.
    e. discount.

42. What is the basic bookkeeping formula?

    a. Charges – payments – adjustments = current balance
    b. Previous balance – charges + payments + adjustments = current balance
    c. Previous balance + charges + payments – adjustments = current balance
    d. Previous balance + charges – payments – adjustments = current balance
    e. Charges – payments + adjustments = current balance

43. Which of the following represents an addition to the balance owed?

    a. Debit
    b. Credit
    c. Payment
    d. Adjustment
    e. Previous balance

44. Which of the following represents a reduction to the balance owed?

    a. Debit
    b. Credit
    c. Payment
    d. Adjustment
    e. Previous balance

45. At the end of each day, you must perform this function to save that day's totals to the month. What is this function called?

    a. Purging
    b. Saving
    c. System backup
    d. Posting
    e. Copying

46. When the current balance is in brackets, this represents a/an:

    a. underpayment.
    b. balance due.
    c. credit balance.
    d. past due balance.
    e. error.

47. Which of the following adjustments reduces the balance owed on an account?

    a. Negative adjustment
    b. Charge
    c. Credit adjustment
    d. Reverse payment
    e. Debit adjustment

48. Which of adjustments increases the balance owed on an account?

    a. Positive adjustment
    b. Payment
    c. Credit adjustment
    d. Reserve charge
    e. Debit adjustment

49. When the office receives an NSF, which of the following steps should you take?

    a. Credit adjustment for the amount of the check, charge office NSF fees, and contact patient.
    b. Debit adjustment for the amount of the check, charge office NSF fees, and contact the patient.
    c. Charge the amount of the check plus office NSF fees and contact the patient.
    d. Charge the amount of the check, debit adjustment for the office NSF fees, and contact the patient.
    e. Send the NSF check directly to the prosecuting attorney's office.

50. Money owed by the office to others is called:

    a. accounts receivable.
    b. receivable accounts.
    c. accounts payable.
    d. accounts adjustable.
    e. cycle accounts.

51. Money patients owe to the office is referred to as:

    a. accounts receivable.
    b. payable accounts.
    c. accounts payable.
    d. accounts adjustable.
    e. cycle accounts.

52. The act of balancing the office checking account is called:

    a. overdrafting.
    b. endorsement.
    c. posting.
    d. reconciliation.
    e. credit balancing.

53. A _____, attached to the deliver, is always used to check actual contents received.

    a. order form
    b. inventory sheet
    c. supply slip
    d. purchase order
    e. packing slip

54. Once supplies are received and verified, the packing slip is saved until the bill or _____ arrives and is checked for accuracy.

    a. receiving slip
    b. purchase order
    c. invoice
    d. inventory sheet
    e. supply slip

55. What is the name of the small fund that is kept on hand to make small purchases for the office?

    a. Accounts payable
    b. Emergency fund
    c. Petty cash
    d. Accounts receivable
    e. Purchase fund

56. Which of the following represent federal taxes that are withheld from employees' paychecks?

    a. FIT, FICA, and Medicare
    b. FICA, Medicare, and Medicaid
    c. FICA, SS, and Medicare
    d. FIT and SS
    e. FIT and Medicare

57. Employees must complete this form declaring the number of dependents they want to claim. This form is called:

    a. W2.
    b. FICA.
    c. FIT.
    d. W4.
    e. I9.

58. To calculate the federal withholdings from an employee's paycheck, you must know the employee's:

    a. pay schedule, amount of pay, marital status, and number of claimed dependents.
    b. salary, marital status, and number of claimed dependents.
    c. pay schedule, amount of pay, and number of claimed dependents.
    d. amount of pay and number of claimed dependents.
    e. pay schedule and amount of pay.

59. Which of the following is used to calculate the exact amount of federal taxes to withhold from an employee's check?

    a. State tax tables
    b. 1,040 tax tables
    c. W2
    d. W4
    e. IRS tax tables

60. Which of the following represents the amount the office must pay for FICA and Medicare taxes on each employee?

    a. Amount withheld from the employees paychecks
    b. Amount withheld from the employees paychecks plus an amount equal to that for the employer contribution
    c. Amount withheld from the employees paychecks plus 50% of that amount as the employer contribution
    d. Amount withheld for the employees paychecks plus 25% of that amount as the employer contribution
    e. Amount withheld for the employees paychecks plus $150 as the employer contribution

61. Employers are also required to pay a quarterly unemployment tax. This tax is referred to as:

    a. FIT.
    b. SS.
    c. FICA.
    d. Medicare.
    e. FUTA.

62. If a patient had a previous balance of $300, then was seen and charged $125, made a payment of $100, and an insurance payment was received in the $150 with the nonallowable portion equaling $50, what is the patient's current balance?

    a. $725
    b. $425
    c. $25
    d. $225
    e. $125

BRIEF EXPLANATIONS

63. Explain how RBRVS and UCR guide the way an office structures its fees.

    _____

    _____

    _____

    _____

64. Describe steps you can take to generate good collection practices.

    _____

    _____

    _____

    _____

65. List three types of payments typically accepted in the medical office. Which method(s) offer the best option(s) to the office?

_____

_____

_____

_____

66. Explain when and why adjustments used.

_____

_____

_____

_____

67. List three items that create expense when billing patients.

_____

_____

_____

_____

68. List four changes that might occur to a patient's account from one billing period to the next.

_____

_____

_____

_____

WHAT DO YOU DO?

69. Read the following scenario and respond to the questions with a short answer.

A patient that is being seen today has written two NSF checks to the office in the past. She has cleared the account and understands that you must pay for all future visits with cash, debit, or credit card. When she arrived, she paid her co-payment in cash. The physician has ordered labs on the patient.

a. How can you check her financial responsibility after insurance?

_____

_____

_____

_____

b. If the patient owes a large amount of money and is unable to pay at the time of service, would you extend an offer of credit (something your office has done for other patients)?

_____

_____

_____

_____

c. Should you allow the NSF checks affect your extension of credit?

_____

_____

_____

_____

d. If she agrees to the offer of credit, what steps would you take to ensure terms are understood and committed too?

_____

_____

_____

_____

PATIENT EDUCATION

70. Write a short narrative script that you can use to provide patient education explaining the billing practice of your office.

_____

_____

_____

_____

INTERNET RESEARCH

Visit the AAPC Web site at https://www.aapc.com and search best billing practices. Select a blog/article to review. Discuss information that you found to be useful in the medical office.

_____

_____

_____

_____

_____

_____

Procedure 13-1   Posting Charges, Payments, and Adjustments

Name: _____   Date: _____   Time: _____   Grade: _____

Equipment: Computer system equipped with medical practice accounting software, current fee schedule, completed encounter forms, and current coding books (ICD, CPT, and HCPCS)

Performance Requirement: Student will perform this skill with ____% accuracy not to exceed _____ minutes. (Instructor will determine the point value for each step, % accuracy, and minutes required.)

Performance Checklist

Point Value	Performance Points Earned	Procedure Steps
		1. Log into the practice accounting software and ensure that the current date appears on charge entry screen.
		2. As patients check out, verify that all billing and insurance information was updated at check in.
		3. Enter each procedure, using the appropriate code for service, and charge (or verify charge if automatic).
		4. Calculate patient's responsibility and collect this amount (or if collected at check in, ensure that it is applied to current charges).
		5. Enter the payment type and payment amount using appropriate payment codes.
		6. Save the changes made to the patient's account.
		7. Offer the patient a receipt, print the receipt, and explain that the remaining balance will be sent to insurance for processing. Be sure they understand any remaining balance following insurance payment will be their responsibility.
		8. Once payment is received from insurance, post the payment (using the appropriate payment code) using the EOB as your guide.
		9. Calculate the amount of the adjustment (amount charge – allowable fee). Enter this amount as an adjustment to the account.
		10. Bill for any remaining balance.

(Continued)

Procedure 13-1 | **Posting Charges, Payments, and Adjustments (*Continued*)**

CALCULATION

Total Points Possible: _____

Total Points Earned: _____

Points Earned/Points Possible = _____%

Student completion time (minutes): _____

PASS   FAIL   COMMENTS:

_____

Student's signature _____   Date _____

Instructor's signature _____   Date _____

Procedure 13-2   Managing Accounts in Collection

Name:: _____ Date: _____ Time: _____ Grade: _____

Equipment: Computer with medical practice accounting software, collection agency data sheets, and listing of delinquent accounts.

Performance Requirement: Student will perform this skill with ____% accuracy not to exceed _____ minutes. (Instructor will determine the point value for each step, % accuracy, and minutes required.)

Performance Checklist

Point Value	Performance Points Earned	Procedure Steps
		1. Determine which accounts will be sent to the collection agency.
		2. Adjust each account individually. Each account will have an adjustment equal to the total balance being sent to collection. Tag the account as Collections so no new charges will be allowed.
		3. Gather all necessary information from each account, to include all billing information and the amount of each account. Submit this information to the collection agency.
		4. As payments are received on a collection account, a reverse or credit adjustment will need to be made. The adjustment should only be for the amount of the payment.
		5. Once the reverse adjustment has been made and the account shows a balance equal to the amount of the payment, post the payment as a collection payment.

CALCULATION

Total Points Possible: _____

Total Points Earned: _____

Points Earned/Points Possible = _____%

Student completion time (minutes): _____

PASS   FAIL   COMMENTS:

_____

Student's signature _____ Date _____

Instructor's signature _____ Date _____

Procedure 13-3 — Processing an NSF (Nonsufficient Funds) Check

Name:: _____ Date: _____ Time: _____ Grade: _____

Equipment: Computer with medical practice accounting software, NSF check, and posted signage of fees charged for returned checks.

Performance Requirement: Student will perform this skill with ____% accuracy not to exceed _____ minutes. (Instructor will determine the point value for each step, % accuracy, and minutes required.)

Performance Checklist

Point Value	Performance Points Earned	Procedure Steps
		1. Upon receipt of the NSF check, first post the amount of the check back to the appropriate account using a reverse or credit adjustment.
		2. Enter a charge for the returned check fee. This is entered as a charge as it is a new fee to this account.
		3. Contact the patient by phone notifying them of the returned check and fees charged. Make arrangements for payment in full. Set a clear deadline.
		4. If unable to reach the patient by phone, send them a certified letter with return receipt explaining the situation. Give a clear deadline as to when the payment is due in the office to avoid further action.
		5. When payment is received (cash, debit, or credit card only), post to the account as a payment. Note that the payment is for NSF plus fees.
		6. If payment is not received timely, the check can be sent to the prosecuting attorney's office in your area for collection or your office can send the account to a collection agency.

CALCULATION

Total Points Possible: _____

Total Points Earned: _____

Points Earned/Points Possible = _____%

Student completion time (minutes): _____

PASS   FAIL   COMMENTS:

_____

Student's signature _____ Date _____

Instructor's signature _____ Date _____

| Procedure 13-4 | Reconciling the Office Bank Statement | |

Name: _____ Date: _____ Time: _____ Grade: _____

Equipment: Bank statement, reconciliation worksheet, checkbook ledger, ending balance of previous bank statement, calculator, and pen.

Performance Requirement: Student will perform this skill with _____% accuracy not to exceed _____ minutes. (Instructor will determine the point value for each step, % accuracy, and minutes required.)

Performance Checklist

Point Value	Performance Points Earned	Procedure Steps
		1. Compare the opening balance on current bank statement with the closing balance of the previous bank statement.
		2. Check the bank statement for service fees, withdraws, and automatic payments. Ensure these all appear on the ledger. If any are missing from the ledger, make an entry noting the date and amount then subtract from the ledger balance (this will be your current balance). Enter the current balance of the account, from the checkbook ledger, on the reconciliation form.
		3. Compare check entries on the bank statement with the ledger. Place a check mark by each cleared check, and be sure to verify that check amounts are the same.
		4. Record any checks not cleared by the bank that appear on the ledger (those without check marks).
		5. Add the amount of all outstanding checks and record the total on the reconciliation form.
		6. Compare all deposits listed on the bank statement with those on the ledger. Place a check mark by each deposit that appears on both.
		7. Record any outstanding deposits that are listed on the ledger, however, are not listed on the bank statements on the reconciliation form.
		8. Total the outstanding deposits.
		9. Add the total of outstanding checks to the starting balance.
		10. Subtract the total of any outstanding deposits from the balance.
		11. The balance on the reconciliation sheet should match the balance on the bank statement.
		12. If the balance do not match, double-check your math first. Then, repeat the process to ensure that you haven't missed any fees, checks, or deposits.

(Continued)

Procedure 13-4 Reconciling the Office Bank Statement (*Continued*)

CALCULATION

Total Points Possible: _____

Total Points Earned: _____

Points Earned/Points Possible = _____%

Student completion time (minutes): _____

PASS   FAIL   COMMENTS:

_____

Student's signature _____   Date _____

Instructor's signature _____   Date _____

14 Health Insurance and Processing Claims

Chapter Objectives

- Describe the differences between group, individual, and government-sponsored health benefit plans.
- Explain the difference between Medicare and Medicaid.
- Explain how managed care programs work.
- Point out similarities and differences between HMOs and PPOs.
- Apply third-party guidelines.
- Apply managed care policies and procedures.
- Summarize how to file claims with Medicare, Medicaid, workers' compensation, and private insurance.
- Complete insurance claim forms.

CAAHEP & ABHES Competencies

CAAHEP

- Identify types of third-party plans.
- Demonstrate understanding of information required to file a third-party claim.
- Identify the steps for filing a third-party claim.
- Outline managed care requirements for patient referral.
- Describe processes for verification of eligibility for services.
- Describe processes for precertification and preauthorization.
- Define a patient-centered medical home (PCMH).
- Differentiate between fraud and abuse.
- Interpret information on an insurance card.

ABHES

- Process insurance claims.
- Differentiate between procedures of private, federal, and state payers.
- Understand the differences between HMO, PPO, and IPA managed care programs.
- Explain the process for obtaining referrals and precertification.

TERMINOLOGY MATCHING

Directions: Match the terms in Column A with the definitions in Column B.

Column A

Column B

1. _____ Assignments of benefits

2. _____ Balance billing

3. _____ Birthday rule
4. _____ Clearinghouse

5. _____ Coinsurance

6. _____ Coordination of benefits
7. _____ Co-payment

8. _____ Crossover claim

9. _____ Deductible
10. _____ Dependents
11. _____ Gatekeeper
12. _____ Medicaid
13. _____ Medicare

14. _____ Medigap
15. _____ Participating provider

16. _____ Preauthorization

17. _____ Precertification
18. _____ Preexisting conditions
19. _____ Referrals
20. _____ Third-party administrator

21. _____ TRICARE

22. _____ Utilization management

23. _____ Utilization review

a. Determines the primary plan when two parents insure a child based on the parent whose birthday occurs first during the year
b. Determines each insurance company's responsibility when a patient has more than one insurance
c. Coordinates the patients' care
d. The patient allows the insurance company to send payments directly to the physician
e. When the unpaid amount of a Medicare claim is automatically transmitted to Medicaid
f. Injuries or illnesses the patient had before the policy took effect
g. Evaluation of medical necessity weighing the costs of care to the benefits
h. A company that provides electronic submission and translation services between doctor offices and insurance companies
i. A health benefits plan for persons aged 65 years and over
j. The provider is in-network
k. A set payment amount that a patient pays per visit
l. Spouse and minor children
m. A health assistance program funded by both federal and state governments
n. The amount the patient must pay before insurance begins to pay
o. Money a patient must pay as his or her share of the cost of treatment
p. Practice of billing the patient for the difference between the physician's usual charge and the health plan's allowable charge
q. Often required before performance of expense testing
r. Policies cover amounts not covered by original Medicare
s. Also referred to as Utilization Management
t. When an employer hires an insurance company or other company to review claims and make payment from the employer's funds
u. Approval to see a specialist is given by the insurance at the recommendation of the PCP
v. Review of patients' care based on diagnoses and cost management
w. A government program sponsored by the U.S. Department of Defense

DEFINING ABBREVIATIONS

Directions: Provide the specific meaning of each of the following abbreviations. Watch your spelling.

24. CHAMPVA: _____

_____

25. EOB: _____

_____

26. EPO: _____

_____

27. HDHP: _____

_____

28. HMO: _____

_____

29. PCP: _____

_____

30. POS: _____

_____

31. PPO: _____

_____

32. UM: _____

_____

33. UR: _____

_____

MAKING IT RIGHT

Each of the following statements is false. Rewrite the statement to make it a true statement.

34. Group insurance plans can be purchased through an insurance broker or from a State Marketplace.

_____

_____

_____

_____

35. A Medigap policy covers services, deductibles, and coinsurance not covered by Medicaid. This policy covers the balance remaining after Medicaid pays a claim.

_____

_____

_____

_____

36. Patients with HDHP pay high monthly payments but have low annual deductibles.

_____

_____

_____

_____

37. The birthday rule applies when both parents have insurance on a child. According to the rule, the oldest parent's insurance is primary.

_____

_____

_____

_____

38. When a patient signs to allow the assignment of benefits, all payments go directly to the patient.

_____

_____

_____

_____

MULTIPLE CHOICE

Directions: Choose the best answer for each question.

39. When an employer has a self-funded plan, they are referred to as a:

    a. participating provider.
    b. third-party payer.
    c. preferred provider.
    d. third-party administrator.
    e. primary administrator.

40. Which of the following represent the government health plan that covers individual aged 65 years and older?

    a. Medicare
    b. Medicaid
    c. TRICARE
    d. CHAMPUS
    e. CHIP

41. When a patient has an illness prior to the start of his or her insurance policy, it is referred to as a:

    a. liability.
    b. preexisting condition.
    c. coordination of benefits.
    d. acute condition.
    e. chronic condition.

42. Which of the following represent the government health plan that covers the families of active duty military members?

    a. Medicare
    b. Medicaid
    c. TRICARE
    d. CHAMPVA
    e. CHIP

43. Which of the following government health plans is design to meet the health care needs of children up to the age of 19 whose family income is too high to qualify for other assistance programs?

    a. Medicare
    b. Medicaid
    c. TRICARE
    d. CHAMPVA
    e. CHIP

44. A payment from any source other than the patient/guarantor is referred to as a\an:

    a. liability case.
    b. HMO.
    c. third-party payer.
    d. PPO.
    e. EPO.

45. Which of the following requires a gatekeeper?

    a. PPO
    b. HDHP
    c. POS
    d. HMO
    e. EPO

46. A gatekeeper coordinates the patients' care and is also referred to as the:

    a. PPO.
    b. consultant.
    c. specialist.
    d. PCP.
    e. HMO.

47. The amount a patient must pay in medical expenses before his or her insurance will start paying:

    a. coinsurance.
    b. deductible.
    c. coordination of benefits.
    d. contracted expenses.
    e. penalty.

48. A Medicare patient is seen in the office today, which of the below covers physician/outpatient expenses?

    a. Part A
    b. Part B
    c. Part C
    d. Part D
    e. Part F

49. Which of the below would cover a Medicare patient's hospital bills?

    a. Part A
    b. Part B
    c. Part C
    d. Part D
    e. Part F

50. Medicare Part D would cover which of the following expenses?

    a. Inpatient hospital care
    b. Medical office visit
    c. Cost of medications
    d. Laboratory tests
    e. Mammogram

51. Precertification is sometimes called:

    a. preregistration.
    b. claim management.
    c. crossover claim.
    d. coordination of benefits.
    e. utilization management.

52. A preset dollar amount the patient owes for each office visit is termed a/an:

    a. deductible.
    b. coinsurance.
    c. coordination of benefits.
    d. assignment of benefits.
    e. co-payment.

53. If a provider is in-network, they are referred to as a:

    a. primary care provider.
    b. non-participating provider.
    c. referring provider.
    d. participating provider.
    e. premier provider.

54. If a patient elects to see an out-of-network provider, which of the following will occur?

    a. The patient will have higher out of pocket expense.
    b. The insurance company will increase the premiums the patient pays.
    c. The patient will have lower out of pocket expense.
    d. Insurance will cover the entire cost of care.
    e. The physician will share the cost of care.

55. When a patient has an EPO and uses an out-of-network provider, which of the following is true?

    a. No benefits will be paid by the insurance company.
    b. Insurance will only pay 50% of the UCR fee.
    c. Full benefits will be paid by the insurance company.
    d. Patient's deductible is waved.
    e. Patient's co-payment is $100.

56. Which of the following applies to a POS plan?

    a. A PCP is not required.
    b. The plan operates like a PPO.
    c. Referrals are required for the patient to see a specialist.
    d. Out-of-network providers are covered under the plan.
    e. There are no co-payments or coinsurance fees.

57. The practice of billing the patient for the difference between the physician's usual charge and the health plan's allowable charge is referred to as:

    a. budget billing.
    b. balance billing.
    c. coordination of benefits.
    d. Medigap.
    e. third-party billing.

58. When a claims administrator settles a claim, it sends an/a _____, itemizing the resulting payment.

    a. coordination of benefits
    b. explanation of benefits
    c. statement of benefits
    d. assignment of benefits
    e. billing statement

59. John came into the office with a worker-related injury. How long do you have to submit the First Report of Injury?

    a. 3 days
    b. 24 hours
    c. 48 hours.
    d. 1 week
    e. 72 hours

60. A PAR provider is required to:

    a. bill the patient for anything over the Medicare fee schedule.
    b. participate in balance billing.
    c. participate in all Medigap plans.
    d. agree to Medicare's fee schedule.
    e. adjust any remaining balance after Medicare's payment.

61. The best practice for assuring that you have complete and correct insurance information for each patient is to:

    a. scan the front of the insurance card.
    b. scan the patient's driver's license.
    c. scan the patient information form.
    d. scan the back of the insurance card.
    e. scan the front and back of the insurance card.

62. Which of the following is true regarding a PPO plan?

    a. The patient can choose to see any physician in any specialty at any time.
    b. A PCP is required.
    c. The patient must select a gatekeeper before the insurance can be used.
    d. A referral is required to see a specialist.
    e. Benefits will only be paid for in-network providers.

BRIEF EXPLANATIONS

63. Explain how the birthday rule is applied.

_____

_____

_____

_____

64. List four services that are covered by the state under Medicaid.

_____

_____

_____

_____

65. List four services that would be covered under Medicare Part B.

_____

_____

_____

_____

66. Explain the differences between TRICARE and CHAMPVA.

_____

_____

_____

_____

67. Describe the three general groups of insurance.

_____

_____

_____

_____

68. List the four common types of plans offered by both individual policies and group plans.

_____

_____

_____

_____

WHAT DO YOU DO?

69. Read the following scenario and respond to the questions with a short answer.

Sally is a patient under the care of Dr. Jones. She is scheduled for an office visit next week and you notice her referral will expire the day before her visit. Sally has an HMO that requires referrals for visits to a specialist.

a. What should you do first?

_____

_____

_____

_____

b. Why is the referral important?

_____

_____

_____

_____

c. What steps can you take to ensure that the referral is completed before the visit? If the referral is not completed in time for the visit, what action should be taken?

_____

_____

_____

_____

d. What information will the PCP need from you?

_____

_____

_____

_____

PATIENT EDUCATION

70. Write a short narrative script that you can use when calling to request a precertification of a procedure.

_____

_____

_____

_____

INTERNET RESEARCH

Visit the CMS Web site at https://www.cms.gov and search Medicare Managed Care Appeals and Grievances. After reading through the protocols give a brief summary of how to appeal a denied claim.

_____

_____

_____

_____

_____

_____

_____

Procedure 14-1 | Obtaining Preauthorization for Services

Name: _____ Date: _____ Time: _____ Grade: _____

Equipment: Computer with access to the patient's EHR, telephone or secure Internet, CPT for procedure to be performed, date of service, location of service, physician's name, and tax identification number.

Performance Requirement: Student will perform this skill with ____% accuracy not to exceed _____ minutes. (Instructor will determine the point value for each step, % accuracy, and minutes required)

Performance Checklist

Point Value	Performance Points Earned	Procedure Steps
		1. Locate the appropriate phone number or Web site (typically found on the patient's insurance card) to begin the preauthorization request. Call or access the Web site.
		2. Provide complete details of the procedure or service to be performed including date, time, physician information, CPT code with detailed information about the procedure, and information regarding past treatments the patient has received.
		3. After providing all necessary information, either by phone or computer, wait for the approval authorization or denial. If denied, obtain information regarding the appeals process.
		4. If approved, notify the patient proceed with the procedure or service. If declined, notify the patient and cancel the procedure or service. Inform the physician to see if he/she wants to move forward with an appeal.

CALCULATION

Total Points Possible: _____

Total Points Earned: _____

Points Earned/Points Possible = _____%

Student completion time (minutes): _____

PASS   FAIL   COMMENTS:

_____

Student's signature _____ Date _____

Instructor's signature _____ Date _____

Section IV

Clinical Medical Assistant Skills

15 | Medical Asepsis and Infection Control

Chapter Objectives

- Describe the conditions that help microorganisms live and grow.
- Explain the chain of infection process.
- List different ways that microorganisms are transmitted.
- Describe how the immune system works to fight infection by microorganisms.
- Compare the three levels of infection control and their effectiveness.
- Explain the concept of medical asepsis.
- Perform handwashing.
- Demonstrate knowledge of OSHA guidelines for risk management in the medical office.
- List the components of an exposure control plan.
- Practice standard precautions.
- Identify situations when personal protective equipment should be worn.
- Demonstrate how to use and remove personal protective equipment.
- Prepare and maintain examination and treatment areas.
- Dispose of biohazardous materials.
- Explain the facts about the transmission and prevention of HBV and HIV in the medical office.
- Describe how to avoid becoming infected with HBV and HIV.

CAAHEP & ABHES Competencies

CAAHEP

- Participate in training on standard precautions.
- Practice standard precautions.
- Select appropriate barrier/personal protective equipment (PPE) for potentially infectious situations.
- Perform handwashing.
- Describe the infection cycle, including the infectious agent, reservoir, susceptible host, means of transmission, portals of entry, and portals of exit.
- Define asepsis.

- Identify personal safety precautions as established by OSHA.
- List major types of infectious agents.
- Compare different methods of controlling the growth of microorganisms.
- Match types and uses of personal protective equipment (PPE).
- Discuss the application of standard precautions with regard to all body fluids, secretions, and excretions, blood, nonintact skin, and mucous membranes.

ABHES

- Infection control.
- Biohazards.

TERMINOLOGY MATCHING

Directions: Match the terms in Column A with the definitions in Column B.

Column A

1. _____ Aerobe
2. _____ Anaerobe
3. _____ Antibody
4. _____ Asepsis
5. _____ Bacteria

6. _____ Contagious

7. _____ Contaminated
8. _____ Disinfection
9. _____ Fungi
10. _____ Immunity
11. _____ Microorganisms
12. _____ Normal flora
13. _____ Pathogen

14. _____ Protozoa
15. _____ Resistance

16. _____ Sanitization
17. _____ Sterilization
18. _____ Vector
19. _____ Viable

20. _____ Virus

Column B

a. Diseases are those that can spread easily from one person to another
b. Tiny living things that are too small to see without a microscope
c. A condition in which there are no living pathogens
d. Microbe capable of causing disease
e. Tiny one-celled creatures found in soil or water or on other organisms
f. Tiny bits of protein-coated nucleic acid that invade and take over cells in other living organisms
g. A type of plant organism
h. Organisms that normally live in your body
i. Tiny parasites that live in or on another organism
j. Refers to how well the human body fights disease
k. Microbes that need oxygen to survive
l. A structure that are designed to attack specific pathogens
m. An object that contains pathogens capable of indirect transmission of disease
n. Cleaning items using soap or detergent
o. Destroys all forms of microorganisms, including bacterial spores
p. Microbes that do not need oxygen to survive
q. Refers to the body's ability to fight specific pathogens
r. Alive—capable of living
s. A condition where something that has been touched by a source of pathogens
t. The destruction of pathogens by direct exposure to chemical or physical agents

DEFINING ABBREVIATIONS

Directions: Provide the specific meaning of each of the following abbreviations. Watch your spelling.

21. CDC: _____

_____

22. EPA: _____

_____

23. HEP B: _____

_____

24. HBV: _____

_____

25. HIV: _____

_____

26. OPIM: _____

_____

27. OSHA: _____

_____

28. PPE: _____

_____

29. SDS: _____

_____

30. TB: _____

_____

MAKING IT RIGHT

Each of the following statements is false. Rewrite the statement to make it a true statement.

31. Bacterial infections are capable of spreading to others, and viruses are incapable of transmission from one person to another.

_____

_____

_____

_____

32. The four main groups of pathogens are bacteria, viruses, fungi, and microorganisms.

_____

_____

_____

_____

33. In order to thrive and grow, bacteria require moisture, proper temperature, nutrients, and sunlight.

_____

_____

_____

_____

34. Chronic infections start quickly and last a short time while acute infections may last a lifetime.

_____

_____

_____

_____

35. The Occupational Safety and Health Administration is responsible for ensuring the safety of all patients in health care facilities.

_____

_____

_____

_____

MULTIPLE CHOICE

Directions: Choose the best answer for each question.

36. Protective protein capsules that some bacteria form around them, like a coat of armor, are:

    a. viruses.
    b. spores.
    c. nonpathogenic.
    d. aerobes.
    e. protozoa.

37. Which of these is not part of the preferred environment for most microbes to grow?

    a. Darkness
    b. Body temperature
    c. Oxygen
    d. Acid pH
    e. Nutrients

38. Which of these is not one of the body's natural barriers to stop microbes from entering the body?

    a. Intact skin
    b. Tear production
    c. Stomach acid
    d. Coughing
    e. Diarrhea

39. Inflammation is the:

    a. ability of the body to develop antibodies.
    b. increase in the amount of white blood cells in circulation in the body.
    c. first way the body responds to any outside attack.
    d. process of the immune system creating lymphocytes to fight infection.
    e. body's response to a fever.

40. Cold sores and genital herpes are conditions caused by:

    a. viruses.
    b. protozoa.
    c. spores.
    d. bacteria.
    e. parasites.

41. What type of transmission occurs through handshaking?

    a. Pathogenic
    b. Direct
    c. Viable
    d. Vector
    e. Indirect

42. OSHA requires that newly hired medical office employees have bloodborne pathogen training every:

    a. week.
    b. month.
    c. 3 months.
    d. 6 months.
    e. year.

43. Which of the following items is not disposed of in a biohazard waste container?

    a. Soiled dressings
    b. Unused needles
    c. Bandages removed from a patient's wound
    d. Soiled exam table paper
    e. Soiled examination gloves

44. Which of these is the procedure that explains what to do if employees or visitors are exposed to biohazardous materials in the medical facility?

    a. Risk management plan
    b. Incident reporting plan
    c. Exposure control plan
    d. Biohazard contamination plan
    e. Sharps container management plan

45. If an employee wishes not to receive the hepatitis vaccination offered by the employer, the employee must:

    a. sign a declination form.
    b. have duties reassigned.
    c. resign the position.
    d. submit to hepatitis testing.
    e. be terminated by the employer.

46. Which of these diseases is not transmitted through droplets in the air?

    a. Influenza
    b. Measles
    c. Mononucleosis
    d. Pneumonia
    e. Rabies

47. Medical offices can easily kill the hepatitis B virus on surfaces by cleaning with:

    a. diluted bleach solution.
    b. 70% alcohol.
    c. Betadine.
    d. soap and water.
    e. iodine.

48. The purpose of a sharps injury log is to:

    a. manage employee vaccination records.
    b. document accidental needle punctures.
    c. record employee OSHA training.
    d. manage needle and syringe inventory.
    e. document incident reports.

49. The form provided by manufacturers listing specific information about chemical products used in the medical office is:

    a. an incident report.
    b. a package insert.
    c. a safety data sheet.
    d. an instruction sheet.
    e. a requisition.

50. An example of a disease caused by a fungus is:

    a. influenza.
    b. ringworm.
    c. strep throat.
    d. shingles.
    e. impetigo.

51. A disease caused by a protozoa is:

    a. herpes.
    b. psoriasis.
    c. measles.
    d. pneumonia.
    e. malaria.

52. Which of these represents the pH range that microbes require to live and grow?

    a. 6.35 to 6.45
    b. 6.48 to 7.15
    c. 7.35 to 7.45
    d. 7.80 to 8.25
    e. 8.56 to 9.25

53. Which of these is the infection stage when symptoms start to fade?

    a. Acute
    b. Chronic
    c. Declining
    d. Incubation
    e. Prodromal

54. Which of these represents the proper order for removing PPE after completion of a medical procedure?

    a. First, remove the gloves, then the mask, and last the gown.
    b. First, remove the mask, then the gloves, and last the gown.
    c. First, remove the gown, then the mask, and last the gloves.
    d. First, remove the gown, then the gloves, and last the mask.
    e. First, remove the gloves, then the gown, and last the mask.

55. What is the recommended amount of time that the eyes should be flushed under the eyewash station?

    a. 5 minutes
    b. 10 minutes
    c. 15 minutes
    d. 25 minutes
    e. 30 minutes

56. Which of these represents a form of immunity when antibodies pass from the mother to the fetus across the placenta?

    a. Passive acquired natural immunity
    b. Active acquired natural immunity
    c. Passive artificial immunity
    d. Active artificial immunity
    e. Innate immunity

57. Which of these transmits the West Nile virus to humans?

    a. Birds
    b. Cats
    c. Dogs
    d. Mosquitoes
    e. Rodents

58. Which of these tasks do not require wearing gloves?

    a. Drawing blood
    b. Handling used instruments
    c. Removing bagged trash
    d. Giving injections
    e. Cleaning a biohazard spill

59. Individuals who contract hepatitis B may develop:

    a. bacterial infections.
    b. cirrhosis.
    c. pancreatitis.
    d. gastric cancer.
    e. cholecystitis.

60. When using bleach for disinfection, use a ratio of 1 part bleach to:

    a. 2 parts water.
    b. 5 parts water.
    c. 10 parts water.
    d. 15 parts water.
    e. 20 parts water.

BRIEF EXPLANATIONS

61. Provide the specific differences between sanitization, disinfection, and sterilization.

    _____

    _____

    _____

    _____

62. Describe the difference between aerobes and anaerobes.

    _____

    _____

    _____

    _____

63. List three ways to break the links in the infection cycle.

    _____

    _____

    _____

    _____

64. List five natural defenses the human body has to protect itself from disease.

    _____

    _____

    _____

    _____

65. List four signs of inflammation that are in response to infection.

    _____

    _____

    _____

    _____

66. List four reasons why a person reasons why a susceptible host cannot fight off pathogens.

_____

_____

_____

_____

WHAT DO YOU DO?

67. Read the following scenario and respond to the questions with a short answer.

You are drawing blood on a 70-year-old female patient who is diabetic and is having a routine annual physical examination. As you complete the successful phlebotomy procedure, you accidentally poke yourself, through your glove, with the venipuncture needle.

a. What is your immediate response to this situation? What do you do first?

_____

_____

_____

_____

b. What should you say to the patient about this situation if she asks you what happened?

_____

_____

_____

_____

c. What bloodborne diseases might this patient have? Which ones are you concerned about contracting through the needle puncture incident?

_____

_____

_____

_____

d. As a result of this needle puncture, what does your employer need to do?

_____

_____

_____

_____

PATIENT EDUCATION

68. Write a short narrative script that you can use to provide patient education explaining the reasons the patient should keep open wounds dry, clean, and bandaged.

   _____

   _____

   _____

   _____

INTERNET RESEARCH

Visit the Centers for Disease Control and Prevention Web site at www.cdc.gov, and research food outbreaks. Identify a specific outbreak and state what food and specific bacteria caused the outbreak, and what the outcome was for the public.

   _____

   _____

   _____

   _____

   _____

   _____

   _____

Procedure 15-1 Handwashing For Medical Asepsis

Name: _____ Date: _____ Time: _____ Grade:_____

Equipment: Sink, water, soap, and paper towels

Performance Requirement: Student will perform this skill with _____% accuracy not to exceed _____ minutes. (Instructor will determine the point value for each step, % accuracy, and minutes required.)

Performance Checklist

Point Value	Performance Points Earned	Procedure Steps
		1. Remove rings and wristwatch.
		2. Stand close to sink but not touching throughout procedure.
		3. Used paper towel to turn on faucet and dispose of paper towel.
		4. Wet your hands and wrists under warm running water. Use a clean towel to push the soap dispenser.
		5. Scrub the palms of each hand.
		6. Rinse hands and wrists holding the hands below your elbows and wrists.
		7. Clean your nails using an orangewood stick or nail brush to clean under each nail.
		8. Use a clean paper towel to push the soap dispenser, wash and rinse hands again.
		9. Dry your hands gently with a paper towel and use the paper towel to turn off the faucet handles.
		10. Discard the used paper towel and orange stick.
		11. Use a dry paper towel to turn off the faucets.

CALCULATION

Total Points Possible: _____

Total Points Earned: _____

Points Earned/Points Possible = _____%

Student completion time (minutes): _____

PASS   FAIL   COMMENTS:

_____

Student's signature _____ Date _____

Instructor's signature _____ Date _____

Procedure 15-2 | Removing Contaminated Gloves

Name: _____ Date: _____ Time: _____ Grade: _____

Equipment: Gloves, biohazard waste container, sink, water, soap, and paper towels

Performance Requirement: Student will perform this skill with ____% accuracy not to exceed _____ minutes. (Instructor will determine the point value for each step, % accuracy, and minutes required.)

Performance Checklist

Point Value	Performance Points Earned	Procedure Steps
		1. Grasp the glove of your nondominant hand at the palm with the hands pointed down.
		2. Tug the glove toward the fingertips of your nondominant hand.
		3. Slide your nondominant hand out of the glove by rolling the glove against the palm of the dominant hand.
		4. Hold the soiled glove in the palm of your dominant hand.
		5. Slip your bare fingers under the cuff of the glove you are still wearing without touching the outside of the glove.
		6. Stretch the glove of the dominant hand up and away from your hand while turning the glove inside out.
		7. The first glove should be inside the second glove, and the second glove should be inside out.
		8. Discard the gloves without taking them apart, in a biohazard waste bin.
		9. Wash your hands.

CALCULATION

Total Points Possible: _____

Total Points Earned: _____

Points Earned/Points Possible = _____%

Student completion time (minutes): _____

PASS   FAIL   COMMENTS:

_____

Student's signature _____ Date _____

Instructor's signature _____ Date _____

Procedure 15-3 | Cleaning Examination Tables

Name: _____ Date: _____ Time: _____ Grade: _____

Equipment: Gloves, biohazard waste container, sink, water, soap, paper towels, exam table, table paper, and spray disinfectant

Performance Requirement: Student will perform this skill with ____% accuracy not to exceed _____ minutes. (Instructor will determine the point value for each step, % accuracy, and minutes required.)

Performance Checklist

Point Value	Performance Points Earned	Procedure Steps
		1. Apply clean gloves.
		2. Remove soiled exam table paper folding inward.
		3. Dispose of soiled table paper in a biohazard waste bag.
		4. Spray the table with a commercial germicide or diluted bleach solution and wipe with paper towel.
		5. Discard the towels in the biohazard waste bag.
		6. Remove gloves and wash hands.
		7. Apply new examination table paper.

CALCULATION

Total Points Possible: _____

Total Points Earned: _____

Points Earned/Points Possible = _____%

Student completion time (minutes): _____

PASS   FAIL   COMMENTS:

_____

Student's signature _____ Date _____

Instructor's signature _____ Date _____

Procedure 15-4 | Cleaning Biohazard Spills

Name: _____ Date: _____ Time: _____ Grade:_____

Equipment: Gloves, eyewear, gown, shoe covers, biohazard waste bag, sink, water, soap, paper towels, absorbent material, and spray disinfectant

Performance Requirement: Student will perform this skill with _____% accuracy not to exceed _____ minutes. (Instructor will determine the point value for each step, % accuracy, and minutes required.)

Performance Checklist		
Point Value	**Performance Points Earned**	**Procedure Steps**
		1. Apply clean gloves, eyewear, and shoe covers.
		2. Cover spill with absorbent material.
		3. Use paper towels to pick up the spill and absorbent material.
		4. Dispose of paper towels and absorbent material in a biohazard waste bag.
		5. Spray the area with a commercial germicide or diluted bleach solution.
		6. Wipe with disposable paper towels discarding the towels in the biohazard waste bag.
		7. Keeping gloves on, remove any protective eyewear being careful not to touch your face.
		8. Take off the gown or apron and shoe coverings.
		9. Place the biohazard waste bag in the biohazard waste bin.
		10. Take off your gloves and wash your hands.

CALCULATION

Total Points Possible: _____

Total Points Earned: _____

Points Earned/Points Possible = _____%

Student completion time (minutes): _____

PASS   FAIL   COMMENTS:

_____

Student's signature _____ Date _____

Instructor's signature _____ Date _____

Procedure 15-5   Guidelines for Waste Disposal

Name: _____ Date: _____ Time: _____ Grade: _____

Equipment: Sharps container, biohazard waste bag, and biohazard waste container

Performance Requirement: Student will perform this skill with ____% accuracy not to exceed _____ minutes. (Instructor will determine the point value for each step, % accuracy, and minutes required.)

Performance Checklist

Point Value	Performance Points Earned	Procedure Steps
		1. Demonstrate use of sharps container including placing items safely into the container and sealing the container when full.
		2. Identify items that are disposed of in sharps container.
		3. Identify use of biohazard waste bag.
		4. Identify use of biohazard waste container.
		5. Explain storage of sharps container, biohazard waste bags, and biohazard waste containers.
		6. Explain process for waste pickup by outside service.
		7. Wash hands after handling biohazard bags, biohazard containers, and sharps containers.

CALCULATION

Total Points Possible: _____

Total Points Earned: _____

Points Earned/Points Possible = _____%

Student completion time (minutes): _____

PASS   FAIL   COMMENTS:

_____

Student's signature _____ Date _____

Instructor's signature _____ Date _____

Medical History and Patient Assessment

Chapter Objectives

- List the typical information included on a medical history form.
- Explain the use of different techniques used to collect information during a patient interview.
- Explain how to use open-ended and closed-ended questions during a patient interview to obtain information.
- Perform patient screening via telephone and face to face.
- Explain the difference between patient signs and symptoms.
- Explain the difference between a chief complaint and present illness.
- Summarize how to measure and record a patient's height and weight.
- Explain the differences in taking a patient's temperature using the oral, rectal, axillary, and tympanic methods.
- Explain how the body controls temperature and the factors that influence it.
- Describe how to assess and record a patient's respiration.
- Identify body sites used for palpating a pulse.
- Explain how to choose the correct blood pressure cuff size.
- Describe the five phases of Korotkoff sounds.
- Identify the factors that may affect blood pressure.
- Accurately obtain and record vital signs including blood pressure, pulse, temperature, respiration, and pulse oximetry.

CAAHEP & ABHES Competencies

CAAHEP

- Obtain vital signs.
- Apply critical thinking skills in performing patient assessment and care.
- Use language/verbal skills that enable patients' understanding.
- Demonstrate respect for diversity in approaching patients and families.
- Differentiate between subjective and objective information.

ABHES

- Gather and process documents.
- Obtain vital signs, obtain patient history, and formulate chief complaint.

TERMINOLOGY MATCHING

Directions: Match the terms in Column A with the definitions in Column B.

Column A

1. _____ Afebrile
2. _____ Anthropometric
3. _____ Assessment
4. _____ Diagnosis
5. _____ Familial disorder
6. _____ Febrile
7. _____ Hereditary disorder
8. _____ Homeopathic
9. _____ Hyperpyrexia
10. _____ Metabolism
11. _____ Paraphrasing
12. _____ Pyrexia
13. _____ Reflecting
14. _____ Signs
15. _____ Sphygmomanometer
16. _____ Symptoms

Column B

a. Passed from parents to their offspring
b. Tiny doses of substances that would, in normal doses, produce the symptoms of the disease being treated
c. The normal physical and chemical processes that occur inside the body
d. Has a fever
e. Rephrasing what the patient said in your own words
f. Subjective information
g. The process of identifying a disease or illness
h. Physical measurements of the patient's body
i. Objective information
j. Without fever
k. A blood pressure cuff
l. Extremely high temperature, 105°F to 106°F
m. The process of gathering information in order to determine the patient's problem
n. A fever of 102°F or higher (rectally) or 101°F or higher (orally)
o. A problem that is unusually common within a family
p. Repeating back what the patient said, using open-ended statements

DEFINING ABBREVIATIONS

Directions: Provide the specific meaning of each of the following abbreviations. Watch your spelling.

17. BP: _____

_____

18. CC: _____

_____

19. FH: _____

_____

20. Ht: _____

_____

21. P: _____

_____

22. PH: _____

_____

23. PI: _____

_____

24. R: _____

_____

25. ROS: _____

_____

26. T: _____

_____

27. Wt: _____

_____

MAKING IT RIGHT

Each of the following statements is false. Rewrite the statement to make it a true statement.

28. When taking in patient health information, the patient's family should include only those members legally related to the patient.

_____

_____

_____

_____

29. Reflecting is repeating back what the patient said, using closed-ended statements.

_____

_____

_____

_____

30. Signs include subjective information and symptoms are objective information.

_____

_____

_____

_____

31. Assessment measurements include the patient's height and weight.

_____

_____

_____

32. The patient's temperature is the measurement of the external heat produced by the body.

_____

_____

_____

33. The patient's pulse is the beating of the heart as felt in a vein.

_____

_____

_____

_____

34. A rectal temperature of 100.6°F would register as 96.6°F if taken orally.

_____

_____

_____

_____

MULTIPLE CHOICE

Directions: Choose the best answer for each question.

35. Which of these is not a factor that causes a patient's temperature to vary?

   a. Age
   b. Exercise
   c. Illness
   d. Time of day
   e. Height and weight

36. Hyperpyrexia is a term related to the:

   a. blood pressure.
   b. pulse.
   c. respiration.
   d. temperature.
   e. measurements.

37. Which of these is not a common pulse point on the body?

   a. Radial
   b. Femoral
   c. Ulnar
   d. Popliteal
   e. Carotid

38. The interval between each heartbeat is the:

   a. pulse rate.
   b. pulse rhythm.
   c. pulse rate.
   d. pulse count.
   e. pulse ratio.

39. Internal respiration involves:

   a. gas exchange in the pharynx and larynx.
   b. exhaling of waste products from the lungs.
   c. exchanging gases between the blood and cells.
   d. exchange of oxygen in the alveoli.
   e. inhaling oxygen through the bronchi.

40. The muscle most involved in the breathing process is the:

    a. diaphragm.
    b. pectoralis major.
    c. rectus abdominis.
    d. intercostals.
    e. serratus.

41. Difficult or labored breathing is:

    a. hyperpnea.
    b. bradypnea.
    c. dyspnea.
    d. hypoxia.
    e. apnea.

42. Blood pressure reading measurements are:

    a. cubic centimeters of oxygen.
    b. millimeters of mercury.
    c. degrees of mercury.
    d. millimeters of pressure.
    e. cubic millimeters of oxygen.

43. The proper size of a blood pressure cuff should be:

    a. 40% of the length of the arm.
    b. 20% to 30% of the circumference of the arm.
    c. 50% of the length of the upper arm.
    d. 30% to 40% the circumference of the arm.
    e. 40% to 50% of the circumference of the arm.

44. The artery used to obtain a blood pressure is the:

    a. radial artery.
    b. ulnar artery.
    c. median cubital artery.
    d. brachial artery.
    e. popliteal artery.

45. How many phases are involved in the Korotkoff sounds?

    a. 2
    b. 3
    c. 4
    d. 5
    e. 6

46. The diastolic pressure is determined when:

    a. the last sound is heard.
    b. there is a soft tapping sound.
    c. the sound changes to a distinct tapping.
    d. the first loud beat is heard.
    e. the swishing sound is hears.

47. A pulse pressure of 30 is present when the blood pressure is:

    a. 120/70.
    b. 110/65.
    c. 100/70.
    d. 140/90.
    e. 150/100.

48. When a patient moves from a sitting or lying position to a standing position, it may cause a drop in the blood pressure called:

    a. sudden hypotension.
    b. orthostatic hypotension.
    c. elevated hypotension.
    d. static hypotension.
    e. moving hypotension.

49. The primary cause of atherosclerosis is:

    a. high blood pressure.
    b. loss of elasticity of the arterial walls.
    c. a rupture and scarring of the arterial walls.
    d. thickening of the arterial wall due to aging.
    e. a buildup of plaque on the wall of the arteries.

50. Which of these would not be included in the patient's social history?

    a. Vital sign readings
    b. Diet preferences
    c. Tobacco and alcohol use
    d. Exercise program
    e. Sleeping habits

51. A patient with impaired vision or hearing is an example of:

    a. rephrasing a patient's words.
    b. observing body language.
    c. active listening.
    d. communication barrier.
    e. summarizing.

52. Which of these is an example of an open-ended question?

    a. Is this your first visit with our office?
    b. How old are you?
    c. Why did you come to the office today?
    d. Is there a family member with you?
    e. Do you have a fever?

53. Which of these represents a patient's symptom?

    a. Headache
    b. Nausea
    c. Dizziness
    d. 101°F temp
    e. Stomach pain

54. A patient who is 49″ is:

    a. 3 foot 11 inches.
    b. 4 foot 0 inch
    c. 4 foot 1 inch
    d. 4 foot 2 inches
    e. 4 foot 3 inches

55. Which of these represents a febrile patient?

    a. 97.6°F axillary
    b. 99.6°F oral
    c. 99.6°F rectal
    d. 98.6°F tympanic
    e. 97.6°F oral

56. A patient's temperature is controlled by the:

    a. hypothalamus.
    b. thyroid.
    c. cerebellum.
    d. heart.
    e. cerebrum.

57. The course of a fever represents:

    a. the onset of the fever.
    b. how high the fever is.
    c. the return to normal.
    d. how serious the infection is.
    e. how long the fever lasts.

58. A fever-reducing agent is an:

    a. antibiotic.
    b. anti-inflammatory.
    c. analgesic.
    d. antipyretic.
    e. antihistamine.

59. A Doppler is a device used to measure:

    a. internal temperatures.
    b. infant length.
    c. peripheral pulses.
    d. respiratory rate.
    e. blood pressure.

BRIEF EXPLANATIONS

60. Provide an example of two open-ended questions that a medical assistant would ask a new patient.

    1. _____

    2. _____

61. List three barriers to communication with a patient and a way to overcome each of these barriers.

    1. _____

    2. _____

    3. _____

62. Briefly explain the difference between external and internal respiration.

_____

_____

_____

_____

63. Describe the location of each of these pulse points.

Carotid - _____

Apical - _____

Radial - _____

Femoral - _____

Popliteal - _____

Dorsalis pedis - _____

64. Explain the purpose of recording the rate, rhythm, and volume of a pulse.

_____

_____

_____

_____

65. Explain why it is important to obtain the respiratory rate of a patient without their knowledge that it is being performed.

_____

_____

_____

_____

WHAT DO YOU DO?

66. Read the following scenario and respond to the questions with a short answer.

You are completing vital signs for a new patient having a complete physical examination. You obtained the patient's height and weight first and then the TPR, BP. You also review the patient's health history form completed by the patient prior to coming to the office.

a. The patient left the social history section of the history form blank. What are two questions can you ask the patient to complete this section?

_____

_____

_____

_____

b. The patient asks you whether the blood pressure reading of 140/95 is normal. What will you tell the patient?

_____

_____

_____

_____

c. The patient cannot recall the names of the three medications prescribed by his prior physician. What can you ask the patient that will help identify those drugs?

_____

_____

_____

_____

PATIENT EDUCATION

67. Write a short narrative script that you can use to provide patient education explaining why patients need to tell the physician any over-the-counter medications they take.

_____

_____

_____

_____

INTERNET RESEARCH

Visit the National Institutes for Health Web site at www.nih.gov, and research methods for smoking cessation. Include information for providing patient education.

_____

_____

_____

_____

_____

_____

_____

Procedure 16-1   Interviewing the Patient to Obtain a Medical History

Name: _____ Date: _____ Time: _____ Grade: _____

Equipment: Medical history form, black or blue pen.

Performance Requirement: Student will perform this skill with _____% accuracy not to exceed _____ minutes. (Instructor will determine the point value for each step, % accuracy, and minutes required.)

Performance Checklist

Point Value	Performance Points Earned	Procedure Steps
		1. Gather supplies and review the medical history form.
		2. Introduce yourself and explain purpose of the interview.
		3. Interview the patient in a private area maintaining eye contact.
		4. Use appropriate questions and determine chief complaint and present illness.
		5. Maintain professionalism through interview.
		6. Offer answers to the patient's questions.
		7. Explain the process for the medical examination or procedure scheduled for the patient.

CALCULATION

Total points possible: _____

Total points earned: _____

Points earned/points possible = _____%

Student completion time (minutes): _____

PASS   FAIL   COMMENTS:

_____

Student's signature _____ Date _____

Instructor's signature _____ Date _____

Procedure 16-2 | Document a Chief Complaint and Present Illness

Name: _____ Date: _____ Time: _____ Grade: _____

Equipment: Patient's medical record or progress note form, black or blue pen.

Performance Requirement: Student will perform this skill with ____% accuracy not to exceed _____ minutes. (Instructor will determine the point value for each step, % accuracy, and minutes required.)

Performance Checklist

Point Value	Performance Points Earned	Procedure Steps
		1. Review the established patient's medical history form, or if new patient, develop a new form.
		2. Greet the patient by name and escort to the examination room. Use correct identifying method to ensure the patient is the correct one.
		3. Use open-ended questions to determine the patient's chief complaint or present illness.
		4. Document the information gathered onto the patient's progress report form. Include date, time, and your signature.
		5. Use correct medical terminology and approved abbreviations in charting.
		6. Thank the patient and explain any wait time until the physician will be in the examination room.

CALCULATION

Total Points Possible: _____

Total Points Earned: _____

Points Earned/Points Possible = _____%

Student completion time (minutes): _____

PASS   FAIL   COMMENTS:

_____

Student's signature _____ Date _____

Instructor's signature _____ Date _____

Procedure 16-3 | Measuring Oral Temperature Using a Mercury-Free Glass Thermometer

Name: _____ Date: _____ Time: _____ Grade: _____

Equipment: Mercury-free glass thermometer, thermometer sheath, tissue, disposable exam gloves, and biohazard waste container.

Performance Requirement: Student will perform this skill with _____% accuracy not to exceed _____ minutes. (Instructor will determine the point value for each step, % accuracy, and minutes required.)

Performance Checklist

Point Value	Performance Points Earned	Procedure Steps
		1. Gather supplies, wash hands, and put on gloves.
		2. Use tissue to dry the thermometer if stored in disinfectant solution.
		3. Check the thermometer for chips or cracks.
		4. Shake the thermometer down if reading above 94°F.
		5. Place disposable sheath on thermometer.
		6. Greet the patient and explain the procedure asking about any eating or drinking within the last 15 minutes.
		7. Place thermometer under the patient's tongue asking the patient to keep the mouth closed but not to bite down on the thermometer.
		8. Leave thermometer in place 3 to 5 minutes. Wait 3 minutes for afebrile patient and 5 minutes if febrile.
		9. Wear gloves and remove thermometer from the patient's mouth.
		10. Remove the sheath by holding the edge of the sheath with the thumb and forefinger of one hand and pulling down from the open edge over the length of the thermometer to the bulb. The soiled area should now be inside the sheath.
		11. Discard the sheath in a biohazard waste container.
		12. Hold the thermometer at eye level and read where the column of liquid has risen.
		13. Sanitize and disinfect the thermometer according to office policy.
		14. Remove your gloves and then wash your hands.
		15. Record the temperature reading in the patient's medical record.

Procedure 16-3	Measuring Oral Temperature Using a Mercury-Free Glass Thermometer (*Continued*)

CALCULATION

Total Points Possible: _____

Total Points Earned: _____

Points Earned/Points Possible = _____%

Student completion time (minutes): _____

PASS   FAIL   COMMENTS:

_____

Student's signature _____ Date _____

Instructor's signature _____ Date _____

Procedure 16-4 | Measuring a Rectal Temperature

Name: _____ Date: _____ Time: _____ Grade: _____

Equipment: Glass mercury-free rectal thermometer, disposable plastic sheath, tissues, patient drape, disposable exam gloves, biohazard waste container, lubricant, and disinfectant solution.

Performance Requirement: Student will perform this skill with _____% accuracy not to exceed _____ minutes. (Instructor will determine the point value for each step, % accuracy, and minutes required.)

Performance Checklist

Point Value	Performance Points Earned	Procedure Steps
		1. Gather supplies, wash your hands, and put on gloves.
		2. Use tissues to dry the thermometer if it has been stored in a disinfectant solution.
		3. Carefully check the thermometer for chips or cracks.
		4. Check the thermometer reading. Hold the stem at eye level and turn it slowly to see the liquid in the column.
		5. If the reading is above 94°F, shake down the thermometer.
		6. Insert the thermometer into the plastic sheath.
		7. Spread lubricant onto a tissue and then from the tissue onto the sheath of the thermometer.
		8. Greet the patient by name and explain the procedure.
		9. Ensure the patient's privacy by placing the patient in a side-lying position.
		10. Visualize the anus by lifting the top buttock with your nondominant hand.
		11. Gently insert the thermometer past the sphincter muscle.
		12. Release the upper buttock and hold the thermometer in place with your dominant hand for 3 minutes. The thermometer will not stay in place if you do not hold it. Replace the drape to ensure the patient's privacy but do not move your dominant hand.
		13. After 3 minutes, remove the thermometer and sheath. Discard the sheath in a biohazard waste container. You need to remove the sheath before reading the thermometer to get an accurate reading.
		14. Hold the thermometer horizontal at eye level and note the temperature reading.
		15. Give the patient a tissue to wipe away excess lubricant.

Procedure 16-4 Measuring a Rectal Temperature (*Continued*)

Performance Checklist

Point Value	Performance Points Earned	Procedure Steps
		16. Sanitize and disinfect the thermometer. Then, remove your gloves and wash your hands.
		17. Record the temperature reading in the patient's medical record marking it with the letter "R" next to the reading, to show the temperature was taken rectally.

CALCULATION

Total Points Possible: _____

Total Points Earned: _____

Points Earned/Points Possible = _____%

Student completion time (minutes): _____

PASS   FAIL   COMMENTS:

_____

Student's signature _____ Date _____

Instructor's signature _____ Date _____

Procedure 16-5   Measuring an Axillary Temperature

Name: _____ Date: _____ Time: _____ Grade: _____

Equipment: Glass mercury-free oral thermometer, disposable probe cover, tissues, disposable exam gloves, biohazard waste container, and disinfectant solution.

Performance Requirement: Student will perform this skill with _____% accuracy not to exceed _____ minutes. (Instructor will determine the point value for each step, % accuracy, and minutes required.)

Performance Checklist

Point Value	Performance Points Earned	Procedure Steps
		1. Gather supplies, wash your hands, and put on gloves.
		2. Use tissue to dry the thermometer if it has been stored in a disinfectant solution.
		3. Carefully check the thermometer for chips or cracks.
		4. Check the thermometer reading. If the reading is above 94°F, shake down the thermometer.
		5. Insert the thermometer into the probe cover.
		6. Explain the procedure to the patient. Expose the patient's axilla. Do not expose more of the patient's chest or upper body than is necessary. It's important to protect the patient's privacy at all times.
		7. Place the bulb of the thermometer deep in the axilla. Bring the patient's arm down, crossing the forearm over the chest.
		8. Leave the thermometer in place for 10 minutes.
		9. Remove the thermometer and remove the probe cover.
		10. Discard the probe cover in the biohazard waste container.
		11. Hold the thermometer horizontal at eye level and note the temperature reading.
		12. Sanitize and disinfect the thermometer.
		13. Remove your gloves and wash your hands.
		14. Record the temperature reading in the patient's medical record. Be sure to mark an *A* beside it.

Procedure 16-5	Measuring an Axillary Temperature (*Continued*)

CALCULATION

Total Points Possible: _____

Total Points Earned: _____

Points Earned/Points Possible = _____%

Student completion time (minutes): _____

PASS   FAIL   COMMENTS:

_____

Student's signature _____ Date _____

Instructor's signature _____ Date _____

Procedure 16-6 Measuring Temperature Using an Electronic Thermometer

Name: _____ Date: _____ Time: _____ Grade: _____

Equipment: Electronic thermometer with oral or rectal probe, disposable probe cover, lubricant if rectal method, tissues, disposable exam gloves for rectal method, and biohazard waste container.

Performance Requirement: Student will perform this skill with ____% accuracy not to exceed _____ minutes. (Instructor will determine the point value for each step, % accuracy, and minutes required.)

Performance Checklist

Point Value	Performance Points Earned	Procedure Steps
		1. Gather supplies, wash hands, and put on gloves.
		2. Greet the patient by name and explain the procedure.
		3. Choose the most appropriate method (oral, axillary, or rectal). Attach the appropriate probe to the battery-powered temperature unit.
		4. Insert the probe into the probe cover.
		5. Take the patient's temperature waiting for the electronic unit to beep when it senses that the temperature is no longer rising.
		6. Remove the probe from the patient and note the temperature reading on the digital display screen on the unit.
		7. Discard the probe cover in a biohazard container by depressing a button, usually on the end of the probe.
		8. Remove gloves if wearing them and wash your hands.
		9. Record the patient's temperature reading in the medical record. Use the abbreviation for the appropriate method used.

CALCULATION

Total Points Possible: _____

Total Points Earned: _____

Points Earned/Points Possible = _____%

Student completion time (minutes): _____

PASS   FAIL   COMMENTS:

_____

Student's signature _____ Date _____

Instructor's signature _____ Date _____

Procedure 16-7   Measuring Temperature Using a Tympanic Thermometer

Name: _____   **Date:** _____   **Time:** _____   **Grade:** _____

Equipment: Tympanic thermometer, disposable probe covers, and biohazard waste container.

Performance Requirement: Student will perform this skill with ____% accuracy not to exceed _____ minutes. (Instructor will determine the point value for each step, % accuracy, and minutes required.)

Performance Checklist

Point Value	Performance Points Earned	Procedure Steps
		1. Gather supplies and wash your hands.
		2. Greet the patient by name and explain the procedure.
		3. Insert the ear probe into the probe cover.
		4. With your nondominant hand, straighten the patient's ear canal. Place the end of the ear probe in the patient's ear with your dominant hand.
		5. With the ear probe properly placed in the ear canal, press the button on the thermometer. The reading shows on the digital display in about 2 seconds.
		6. Remove the probe and note the reading.
		7. Discard the probe cover in a biohazard waste container.
		8. Wash your hands.
		9. Record the temperature on the patient's record in the same way that you record temperatures for a glass thermometer. Indicate the method used when charting.

CALCULATION

Total Points Possible: _____

Total Points Earned: _____

Points Earned/Points Possible = _____%

Student completion time (minutes): _____

PASS   FAIL   COMMENTS:

_____

Student's signature _____   Date _____

Instructor's signature _____   Date _____

Procedure 16-8 Measuring the Radial Pulse

Name: _____ Date: _____ Time: _____ Grade: _____

Equipment: Watch or clock with second hand.

Performance Requirement: Student will perform this skill with ____% accuracy not to exceed _____ minutes. (Instructor will determine the point value for each step, % accuracy, and minutes required.)

Performance Checklist

Point Value	Performance Points Earned	Procedure Steps
		1. Wash your hands.
		2. Greet the patient by name and explain the procedure.
		3. Position the patient so the arm is relaxed. Support the arm either on the patient's lap or on a table.
		4. Use the index, middle, and ring fingers of your dominant hand to find the radial pulse. The pulse point is located on the patient's thumb side of the wrist.
		5. Press your fingers on the pulse point. Press firmly enough to feel the pulse.
		6. If the pulse is regular, count it for 30 seconds, watching the second hand of your watch. Multiply the number of pulsations by 2 since the pulse is recorded as the number of beats per minute. If the pulse is irregular, count it for a full 60 seconds. Otherwise, the measurement may be inaccurate.
		7. Record the pulse rate in the patient's medical record with the other vital signs. Make a note if the rhythm is irregular and the volume is thready or bounding.

CALCULATION

Total Points Possible: _____

Total Points Earned: _____

Points Earned/Points Possible = _____%

Student completion time (minutes): _____

PASS   FAIL   COMMENTS:

_____

Student's signature _____ Date _____

Instructor's signature _____ Date _____

Procedure 16-9 | Measuring Respirations

Name: _____ Date: _____ Time: _____ Grade: _____

Equipment: Watch or clock with second hand.

Performance Requirement: Student will perform this skill with ____% accuracy not to exceed _____ minutes. (Instructor will determine the point value for each step, % accuracy, and minutes required.)

Performance Checklist

Point Value	Performance Points Earned	Procedure Steps
		1. Wash your hands.
		2. Greet the patient by name.
		3. Observe carefully for the easiest area to assess respirations. Respirations are measured at the same time as the pulse.
		4. After counting the radial pulse, continue to watch the second hand of your watch and begin counting respirations.
		5. If the breathing pattern is regular, count the respiratory rate for 30 seconds. Then multiply by 2. If the pattern is irregular, count for a full 60 seconds. Otherwise, the measurement may be inaccurate.
		6. Record the respiratory rate in the patient's medical record along with the other vital signs. Also, note the rhythm if irregular. Mark down any unusual sounds, such as wheezing.

CALCULATION

Total Points Possible: _____

Total Points Earned: _____

Points Earned/Points Possible = _____%

Student completion time (minutes): _____

PASS   FAIL   COMMENTS:

_____

Student's signature _____ Date _____

Instructor's signature _____ Date _____

Procedure 16-10 | Measuring Blood Pressure

Name: _____ Date: _____ Time: _____ Grade: _____

Equipment: Sphygmomanometer and stethoscope.

Performance Requirement: Student will perform this skill with ____% accuracy not to exceed _____ minutes.
(Instructor will determine the point value for each step, % accuracy, and minutes required.)

Performance Checklist

Point Value	Performance Points Earned	Procedure Steps
		1. Gather supplies and wash your hands.
		2. Greet the patient by name and explain the procedure.
		3. Properly position the patient with the arm supported and the forearm on the lap or a table.
		4. Expose the patient's arm removing clothing that is too bulky or too tight.
		5. Make sure the patient's legs are not crossed. Ask the patient not to talk during the procedure.
		6. Palpate the brachial pulse in the antecubital area.
		7. Center the deflated cuff directly over the brachial artery. The lower edge of the cuff should be 1 to 2 inches above the antecubital area.
		8. Wrap the cuff smoothly and snugly around the arm. Secure the cuff with the Velcro edges.
		9. Hold the air pump in your dominant hand, with the valve between your thumb and forefinger. Turn the valve screw clockwise to tighten it.
		10. Determine a reference point for how far you need to inflate the cuff. While palpating the brachial pulse with your nondominant hand, inflate the cuff. Note the point or number on the dial or glass tube column at which you no longer feel the brachial pulse. This is the reference point for reinflating the cuff when taking the blood pressure.
		11. Deflate the cuff by turning the valve counterclockwise. Wait at least 30 seconds before reinflating the cuff.
		12. Clean the earpieces of the stethoscope with an alcohol wipe. Place the stethoscope earpieces in your ears with the openings pointed slightly forward. Stand about 18 inches from the manometer with the gauge at eye level to reduce the chances of making an error while taking the reading.
		13. Place the diaphragm of the stethoscope against the brachial artery and hold it in place with your nondominant hand.

Procedure 16-10 | Measuring Blood Pressure (*Continued*)

Performance Checklist

Point Value	Performance Points Earned	Procedure Steps
		14. The stethoscope tubing should hang freely without touching or rubbing any part of the cuff.
		15. With your dominant hand, turn the screw near the bulb just enough to close the valve. Inflate the cuff.
		16. Pump the valve bulb to about 30 mm Hg above the number you noted when palpating the brachial artery.
		17. Once the cuff is inflated appropriately, turn the valve counterclockwise. You want to release the air at about 2 to 4 mm Hg per second.
		18. Listen carefully while watching the gauge. Note the point on the gauge at which you hear the first clear tapping sound. This is the systolic sound or Korotkoff phase 1.
		19. Continue to listen and deflate the cuff. When you hear the last sound, note the reading, and quickly deflate the cuff.
		20. The last sound heard is the Korotkoff phase 5 sound. Record this as the diastolic pressure or the bottom number.
		21. Remove the stethoscope earpieces from your ears. Remove the cuff and press any remaining air from the bladder of the cuff.
		22. Put the equipment away and wash your hands.
		23. Record the reading. The systolic pressure is always written as a fraction over the diastolic pressure (e.g., 120/80). Note which arm was used—RA, for right arm, or LA, for left arm. Record the patient's position if other than sitting.

CALCULATION

Total Points Possible: _____

Total Points Earned: _____

Points Earned/Points Possible = _____%

Student completion time (minutes): _____

PASS   FAIL   COMMENTS:

_____

Student's signature _____ Date _____

Instructor's signature _____ Date _____

17 Assisting with the Physical Examination

Chapter Objectives

- Identify the medical assistant's role in assisting with the physical examination.
- List the equipment and supplies needed in the patient examination room.
- Prepare and maintain patient examination and treatment areas.
- Explain the care and use of the equipment and instruments used in a physical examination.
- Describe six examination techniques used during the physical examination.
- Prepare patients for and assist with routine and specialty examinations.
- Describe the basic examination positions and explain their use.
- Understand the sequential process used by the physician to complete a physical examination.
- Explain how the physician evaluates a patient's posture, gait, and reflexes.
- Instruct patients how to recognize cancer warning signs and perform self-examinations of the breasts and testicles.
- List the guidelines for annual examinations, immunizations, and cancer screening.

CAAHEP & ABHES Competencies

CAAHEP

- Assist physician with patient care.
- Apply critical thinking skills in performing patient assessment and care.
- Use language/verbal skills that enable patients' understanding.
- Demonstrate respect for diversity in approaching patients and families.
- Explain the rationale for performance of a procedure to the patient.
- Document patient care.
- Respond to nonverbal communication.

ABHES

- General/physical examination.
- Specialty examination.
- Working with diverse populations.

TERMINOLOGY MATCHING

Directions: Match the terms in Column A with the definitions in Column B.

Column A

1. _____ Accommodation
2. _____ Asymmetry
3. _____ Auscultation
4. _____ Gait
5. _____ Inspection
6. _____ Manipulation
7. _____ Mensuration
8. _____ Ophthalmoscope
9. ___ Otorhinolaryngologist
10. _____ Otoscope
11. _____ Palpation
12. _____ Percussion
13. _____ Speculum
14. _____ Stethoscope
15. _____ Symmetry

Column B

a. A physician who specializes in treating disorders and diseases of the ears, nose, and throat
b. Listening to body sounds
c. Tapping or striking parts of the body with the hand or an instrument to produce sounds
d. Looking at areas of the body to observe physical features
e. Equality of size and shape
f. The ability of the pupils to adjust when focusing on objects at different distances
g. A medical tool used to inspect the interior structures of the eyes
h. An instrument used for listening to body sounds
i. Inequality of size and shape
j. Touching or moving body areas with the fingers or hands
k. The style or way in which a person walks
l. The process of measuring
m. Is a tool designed to allow examiners to investigate body cavities
n. Allows the examiner to see inside the ear canal and inspect the tympanic membrane
o. Moving a body part or joint

DEFINING ABBREVIATIONS

Directions: Provide the specific meaning of each of the following abbreviations. Watch your spelling.

16. CC: _____

_____

17. CPX: _____

_____

18. ECG: _____

_____

19. PERRLA: _____

_____

20. PAP: _____

_____

21. PH: _____

_____

22. PI: _____

_____

23. ROM: _____

_____

24. ROS: _____

_____

MAKING IT RIGHT

Each of the following statements is false. Rewrite the statement to make it a true statement.

25. A tuning fork is used to test neurological reflexes, the nervous system's response to specific stimuli.

_____

_____

_____

_____

26. The otoscope is a medical tool used to inspect the interior structures of the eyes.

_____

_____

_____

_____

27. A gooseneck light is a small light the size and shape of a ballpoint pen.

_____

_____

_____

_____

28. A cervical scraper is a disposable brush made of nylon or plastic with soft bristles at one end used to obtain cells for a Pap smear.

_____

_____

_____

_____

29. Mensuration is the process of moving a body part or joint during a physical examination.

_____

_____

_____

_____

30. In the Sims position, the patient lies on the back with arms at the sides.

_____

_____

_____

_____

MULTIPLE CHOICE

Directions: Choose the best answer for each question.

31. Which of the following positions requires the patient to have his or her feet supported in stirrups?

   a. Fowler's
   b. Dorsal recumbent
   c. Lithotomy
   d. Sims
   e. Supine

32. Which of these areas would the physician examine first during a complete physical examination?

   a. Breasts
   b. Abdomen
   c. Legs
   d. Eyes
   e. Groin

33. What body part does the physician examine in the area of the throat?

   a. Tympanic membrane
   b. Thyroid gland
   c. Sclera
   d. Auricle
   e. Paranasal sinuses

34. Which of these items is not required for examination of the head and neck?

   a. Stethoscope
   b. Penlight
   c. Tongue blade
   d. Laryngeal mirror
   e. Ophthalmoscope

35. Which of these exam methods requires the use of a stethoscope?

   a. Mensuration
   b. Manipulation
   c. Palpation
   d. Percussion
   e. Auscultation

36. During breast examination, the physician will also examine the:

   a. cervical nodes.
   b. inguinal nodes.
   c. parotid nodes.
   d. axillary nodes.
   e. groin nodes.

37. During a male examination, the physician will perform a rectal examination to determine the size of this gland.

    a. Epididymis
    b. Prostate
    c. Scrotum
    d. Hemorrhoid
    e. Vas deferens

38. The physician will evaluate the style or way in which a person walks by observing the patient's:

    a. peripheral pulses.
    b. posture.
    c. gait.
    d. reflexes.
    e. range of motion.

39. Which tendon tests reflexes located around the kneecap area?

    a. Patellar tendon
    b. Biceps tendon
    c. Achilles tendon
    d. Plantar tendon
    e. Triceps tendon

40. At what age should a person begin testing for colon and rectal cancer?

    a. 20
    b. 30
    c. 40
    d. 50
    e. 60

41. Which of these symptoms is not one of the early warning signs of cancer?

    a. Change in bowel habit
    b. Sore does not heal
    c. Indigestion
    d. Difficulty swallowing
    e. Intermittent fever

42. What is the recommendation to give a tetanus booster to a patient?

    a. Every 2 years
    b. Every time there is an injury
    c. Every 10 years
    d. Every 5 years
    e. When a patient requests it

43. Which of these tasks is the responsibility of the medical assistant during a complete physical examination?

    a. Palpate the patient's breasts for lumps.
    b. Perform percussion on the patient's back.
    c. Manipulate the joints to determine range of motion.
    d. Perform mensuration to determine height and weight.
    e. Perform auscultation of the patient's heart and lungs.

44. Which of these instruments is used when evaluating a patient's hearing?

    a. Otoscope
    b. Tuning fork
    c. Reflex hammer
    d. Speculum
    e. Ophthalmoscope

45. The physician who specializes in treating disorders and diseases of the ears, nose, and throat is:

    a. an otorhinolaryngologist.
    b. a pulmonologist.
    c. an otologist.
    d. an internist.
    e. an ophthalmologist.

46. What type of medical assistant is specialized to teach patients to use and care for contact lenses?

    a. Podiatric assistant
    b. Otology assistant
    c. Pulmonary assistant
    d. Ophthalmic assistant
    e. Pediatric assistant

47. A gynecological examination includes:

    a. a Pap smear.
    b. a breast exam.
    c. a rectal exam.
    d. an abdominal exam.
    e. a uterine biopsy.

48. Which of these examination methods only involves visual observation?

    a. Palpation
    b. Mensuration
    c. Manipulation
    d. Inspection
    e. Auscultation

49. When the patient's breasts are of equal size, the physician will note that the breasts are:

    a. asymmetrical.
    b. contoured.
    c. symmetrical.
    d. normal.
    e. large.

50. What examination method involves tapping or striking the body with the fingers?

    a. Palpation
    b. Percussion
    c. Manipulation
    d. Auscultation
    e. Mensuration

51. What method of examination is used to determine the head circumference of an infant?

    a. Inspection
    b. Auscultation
    c. Palpation
    d. Manipulation
    e. Mensuration

52. When helping the physician with a patient during physical examination, the medical assistant should not:

    a. watch for signs that the patient may be uncomfortable.
    b. move the patient's body quickly.
    c. provide a small pillow to help the patient feel more at ease.
    d. drape the patient exposing only the area to be examined.
    e. remain in the room during the examination.

53. Dorsal recumbent position is used:

    a. to take stress off the patient's back.
    b. for patients with breathing difficulties.
    c. to perform a colonoscopy.
    d. examine the spine.
    e. check the patellar tendon reflexes.

54. At what age should an individual have a baseline electrocardiogram?

    a. 20
    b. 30
    c. 35
    d. 40
    e. 45

55. What examination method does the physician use to determine if the patient has a hernia in the groin region?

    a. Auscultation
    b. Mensuration
    c. Palpation
    d. Percussion
    e. Manipulation

56. What position is preferred for breast examination?

    a. Trendelenburg
    b. Prone
    c. Fowlers
    d. Lithotomy
    e. Supine

57. What examination method does the physician use to assess dental hygiene?

    a. Mensuration
    b. Observation
    c. Auscultation
    d. Inspection
    e. Manipulation

58. Soft growths on membrane linings such as those that can grow in the nostrils are:

    a. lesions.
    b. polyps.
    c. swellings.
    d. obstructions.
    e. malignant.

59. What instrument is used to examine the ear canal?

    a. Otoscope
    b. Ophthalmoscope
    c. Tympanic speculum
    d. Laryngeal mirror
    e. Penlight

60. What instruments and supplies are used during examination of the eyes, nose, and mouth?

    a. Otoscope, penlight, nasal speculum
    b. Nasal speculum, otoscope, gloves
    c. Ophthalmoscope, tongue blade, penlight
    d. Stethoscope, tongue blade, gloves
    e. Ophthalmoscope, otoscope, gloves

BRIEF EXPLANATIONS

61. Complete the following chart providing the information requested.

Body Part Examined	Equipment/Supplies Needed	Examination Method(s)
Ears		
Vagina		
Abdomen		
Throat		

62. List at least five (5) basic exam room supplies and the purpose for each.

    _____

    _____

    _____

    _____

63. List three structures, or areas of the body, the physician examines using a stethoscope. Explain why a stethoscope is needed for this type of evaluation.

    _____

    _____

    _____

    _____

64. After a patient examination, provide a list of tasks that the medical assistant does before another patient can be put in that room.

_____

_____

_____

_____

65. List four (4) common tests that are associated with the complete physical examination and explain the medical assistant's role in completion of these tests.

_____

_____

_____

_____

66. What is the main purpose for a mammogram, and what patients should have this examination performed?

_____

_____

_____

_____

WHAT DO YOU DO?

67. Read the following scenario and respond to the questions with a short answer.

Nancy McPherson is a regular patient of the medical office. During her last visit, the physician asked her to schedule an annual physical examination within the next couple of weeks. She calls the office to schedule the appointment for the examination and asks you several questions.

a. What should you tell her when she asks why the annual exam is necessary since she is in periodically throughout the year?

_____

_____

_____

_____

b. How will you respond to her if asked why she needs a blood and urine test also?

_____

_____

_____

_____

c. When she arrives for the appointment, you ask her about allergies and the status of her immunizations. Why is it necessary to ask an adult these questions?

_____

_____

_____

_____

PATIENT EDUCATION

68. Write a short narrative script that you can use to provide patient education explaining the reasons a female patient should maintain a regular schedule for mammograms and Pap smear examinations.

_____

_____

_____

_____

INTERNET RESEARCH

Visit the National Institutes of Health Web site at www.nih.gov, and research testicular cancer. Include information about the number of men diagnosed annually with this type of cancer, the average age of victims, and the expected outcome of this type of cancer.

_____

_____

_____

_____

_____

_____

_____

Procedure 17-1   Cleaning and Preparing the Examination Room

Name: _____ Date: _____ Time: _____ Grade: _____

Equipment: Disposable gloves

Performance Requirement: Student will perform this skill with ____% accuracy not to exceed _____ minutes. (Instructor will determine the point value for each step, % accuracy, and minutes required.)

Performance Checklist

Point Value	Performance Points Earned	Procedure Steps
		1. Wash hands and put on gloves.
		2. Discard disposable waste in appropriate container. This includes exam table paper and patient gowns.
		3. Remove soiled reusable instruments.
		4. Remove gloves and wash hands. Put on new pair of gloves to continue cleaning.
		5. Use paper towels to remove any visible soil from countertops, cabinets, and surfaces in the exam room.
		6. Wipe surfaces with disinfectant. Check protective coverings on equipment, and if soiled, clean them.
		7. Dispose of paper towels in biohazard waste container.
		8. Check exam room supplies and replenish (cotton applicators, tongue blades, patient gowns, instruments).
		9. Set up equipment and supplies for next examination.
		10. Check equipment to ensure it is working (otoscope, ophthalmoscope, lights).
		11. Replace new table paper and proper gown for the next patient.

(Continued)

Procedure 17-1 | **Cleaning and Preparing the Examination Room (*Continued*)**

CALCULATION

Total Points Possible: _____

Total Points Earned: _____

Points Earned/Points Possible = _____%

Student completion time (minutes): _____

PASS   FAIL   COMMENTS:

_____

Student's signature _____ Date _____

Instructor's signature _____ Date _____

Procedure 17-2 | Preparing the Adult Patient for the Physical Examination

Name: _____ Date: _____ Time: _____ Grade: _____

Equipment: Patient medical record

Performance Requirement: Student will perform this skill with ____% accuracy not to exceed _____ minutes. (Instructor will determine the point value for each step, % accuracy, and minutes required.)

Performance Checklist

Point Value	Performance Points Earned	Procedure Steps
		1. Wash hands.
		2. Properly greet and identify the patient. Escort patient to the prepared examination room.
		3. Obtain and record the patient's medical history and chief complaint.
		4. Measure and record the patient's vital signs, height, weight, and visual acuity.
		5. If requested by the physician, instruct the patient to obtain a urine specimen. Direct the patient to the bathroom.
		6. When the patient returns to the examination room, provide instructions for disrobing and explain how to put on the gown, open in the front or back depending on exam performed.
		7. Leave the room unless the patient needs assistance.
		8. When patient is undressed and in the gown, assist patient to sit on the end of the exam table. Cover the patient's legs with a drape.
		9. Enter all information into the patient's medical record. If paper chart is used, place the patient's medical record in a secure location outside the exam room and notify the physician that the patient is ready.

(Continued)

Procedure 17-2 | **Preparing the Adult Patient for the Physical Examination (*Continued*)**

CALCULATION

Total Points Possible: _____

Total Points Earned: _____

Points Earned/Points Possible = _____%

Student completion time (minutes): _____

PASS   FAIL   COMMENTS:

_____

Student's signature _____ Date _____

Instructor's signature _____ Date _____

Procedure 17-3 | **Assisting with Patients in Wheelchairs** PSY

Name: _____ Date: _____ Time: _____ Grade: _____

Equipment: Wheelchair

Performance Requirement: Student will perform this skill with ____% accuracy not to exceed _____ minutes.
(Instructor will determine the point value for each step, % accuracy, and minutes required.)

Performance Checklist

Point Value	Performance Points Earned	Procedure Steps
		1. Wash your hands and greet the patient by name. If necessary, ask another staff member to assist you.
		2. Bring the wheelchair as close as possible to the end of the examination table and place at a 90-degree angle to the table to minimize the distance for moving the patient.
		3. Lock the wheels to stop the wheelchair from moving.
		4. Check to make sure the patient is wearing shoes or slippers with nonskid soles. Lift the patient's feet off the footrests. Fold up the footrests so the patient does not trip over them. Keep your own feet in front of the patient's feet to prevent the patient from slipping.
		5. If you are moving the patient yourself, face the patient and ask the patient to hold onto your shoulders. Your knees should be in line with the patient's knees. Bending your knees slightly will lower your body and make it easier for the patient reach you.
		6. Place your arms under the patient's arms and around the patient's body. Prepare the patient by explaining that you will count to three and then lift. If possible, the patient can help by supporting some of her body weight.
		7. Count to three and lift the patient. Turn toward the examination table. The back of the patient's knees should touch the table.
		8. Lower the patient onto the examination table. If the patient cannot sit without support, help the patient into a supine position. Otherwise, keep the patient in a sitting position.
		9. If someone else is helping you move the patient, decide which one of you will turn the patient toward the examination table during the transfer. The stronger person should perform this maneuver.

(*Continued*)

| Procedure 17-3 | Assisting with Patients in Wheelchairs (*Continued*) |

Performance Checklist

Point Value	Performance Points Earned	Procedure Steps
		10. You and your helper should both face the patient with your knees slightly bent. Each of you should have one knee in line with the patient's knees. The patient will put one hand on each person's shoulder.
		11. Place one of your arms around the patient. Your helper should do the same. Lock your wrists together to provide extra support. On the count of three, lift the patient together.
		12. One person turns the patient toward the examination table, and then, both of you will gradually lower the patient onto the table.
		13. After the patient is comfortable and safely positioned on the examination table, unlock the wheels on the wheelchair and move it back from the table to an area where it will not get in the way.
		14. Provide the patient with a gown and drape. If necessary, help the patient disrobe.

CALCULATION

Total Points Possible: _____

Total Points Earned: _____

Points Earned/Points Possible = _____%

Student completion time (minutes): _____

PASS   FAIL   COMMENTS:

_____

Student's signature _____ Date _____

Instructor's signature _____ Date _____

Procedure 17-4 | Assisting with Pregnant Patients

Name: _____ Date: _____ Time: _____ Grade: _____

Equipment: Patient's medical record

Performance Requirement: Student will perform this skill with ____% accuracy not to exceed _____ minutes.
(Instructor will determine the point value for each step, % accuracy, and minutes required.)

Performance Checklist

Point Value	Performance Points Earned	Procedure Steps
		1. Wash your hands.
		2. Properly greet and identify the patient by name, and escort her to the prepared examining room.
		3. Prepare the patient for the examination as you would for any other adult patient explaining the examination procedure.
		4. Measure and record vital signs, height, and weight.
		5. Instruct the patient on collecting a urine sample. The physician may require a urine test.
		6. Ask the patient if she has any specific questions regarding her pregnancy. Notify the physician of these questions prior to her examination. Provide the patient with education materials that may address her concerns.
		7. Provide instructions for disrobing and explain how to put on the gown. Leave the room to give the patient privacy while disrobing. Ask if she needs any assistance.
		8. Have the patient use a stool to step up to the examining table. Help her sit on the end of the table. Cover her legs with a drape and provide additional drapes as needed for privacy.
		9. During the examination, take care when asking the patient to move into different body positions.
		10. Watch for signs that the patient is uncomfortable. Be especially vigilant during changes in body position.
		11. At the end of the examination, help the patient down from the examination table. Leave the room to give her privacy while she dresses. Ask her if she needs assistance.

(Continued)

Procedure 17-4   Assisting with Pregnant Patients (*Continued*)

CALCULATION

Total Points Possible: _____

Total Points Earned: _____

Points Earned/Points Possible = _____%

Student completion time (minutes): _____

PASS   FAIL   COMMENTS:

_____

Student's signature _____ Date _____

Instructor's signature _____ Date _____

Procedure 17-5   Assisting with the Adult Physical Examination

Name: _____ Date: _____ Time: _____ Grade: _____

Equipment: Patient medical record, examination instruments, and disposable gloves

Performance Requirement: Student will perform this skill with ____% accuracy not to exceed _____ minutes.
(Instructor will determine the point value for each step, % accuracy, and minutes required.)

Performance Checklist

Point Value	Performance Points Earned	Procedure Steps
		1. Wash your hands and prepare the examination room and patient.
		2. When the physician is ready to begin the physical examination, you will assist by handing the physician the appropriate instruments and positioning the patient appropriately.
		3. Help the patient lower the gown to the waist for examination of the chest and upper back. The physician will use a stethoscope during the chest exam.
		4. Help the patient pull up the gown and remove the drape from the legs. Hand the physician the reflex hammer to test patient reflexes.
		5. Help the patient into the supine position. Open the gown at the top to expose the chest again. Place the drape over the waist, abdomen, and legs. The physician will examine the breasts and may again listen to chest sounds.
		6. Cover the patient's chest. Lower the drape to expose the abdomen. The physician will use a stethoscope to listen to bowel sounds.
		7. Prepare and position the patient for examination of the genital and rectal areas.
		8. Position female patients in lithotomy; position male patients according to physician preference for rectal and prostate exam.
		9. Provide tissues to patient following vaginal and rectal exams.
		10. With the patient standing, the physician may assess legs, gait, coordination, and balance.
		11. Help the patient sit on the end of the examination table so the physician can discuss findings with the patient.

(Continued)

Procedure 17-5 | Assisting with the Adult Physical Examination (*Continued*)

Performance Checklist

Point Value	Performance Points Earned	Procedure Steps
		12. Perform or schedule any follow-up procedures or treatments.
		13. Leave the room while the patient dresses unless the patient needs assistance.
		14. Return to the examination room when the patient has dressed to answer any questions, reinforce instructions, and provide patient education.
		15. Escort the patient to the front desk.
		16. Properly clean or dispose of all used equipment and supplies.
		17. Clean the counter surfaces of the room and the examination table with a disinfectant and prepare for the next patient.
		18. Wash your hands and record any instructions from the physician in the patient's record. Note any test results, specimens taken for testing, and the laboratory where the specimens were sent.

CALCULATION

Total Points Possible: _____

Total Points Earned: _____

Points Earned/Points Possible = _____%

Student completion time (minutes): _____

PASS   FAIL   COMMENTS:

_____

Student's signature _____ Date _____

Instructor's signature _____ Date _____

Procedure 17-6 Measuring Distance Visual Acuity

Name: _____ Date: _____ Time: _____ Grade: _____

Equipment: Snellen eye chart, eye occluder, and patient medical record

Performance Requirement: Student will perform this skill with ____% accuracy not to exceed _____ minutes. (Instructor will determine the point value for each step, % accuracy, and minutes required.)

Performance Checklist

Point Value	Performance Points Earned	Procedure Steps
		1. Wash your hands and prepare the examination area. Ensure the area is well lighted.
		2. Identify the patient by name and explain the procedure.
		3. Position the patient at the 20-foot mark. The patient may be standing or sitting, as long as the chart is at eye level.
		4. Note whether the patient is wearing glasses. If not, ask about contact lenses and record the information. Patients usually wear their corrective lenses during the visual acuity examination. The patient record must indicate if the patient is wearing contact lenses or glasses.
		5. Have the patient cover the left eye with an eye occluder. Instruct the patient to keep both eyes open, even though one is covered.
		6. Stand beside the eye chart, point to each row as the patient reads it aloud. Begin with the 20/200 line. If the patient can read these lines easily, move down to smaller figures.
		7. Record the smallest line the patient can read with no more than one error or according to office policy. Record the eye tested, the line number, and the errors.
		8. Repeat the procedure with the right eye covered.
		9. Repeat step 7 with both eyes uncovered. Record the results using the abbreviation for both eyes, OU.
		10. Document the procedure in the patient's record.

(Continued)

Procedure 17-6   Measuring Distance Visual Acuity (*Continued*)

CALCULATION

Total Points Possible: _____

Total Points Earned: _____

Points Earned/Points Possible = _____%

Student completion time (minutes): _____

PASS   FAIL   COMMENTS:

_____

Student's signature _____   Date _____

Instructor's signature _____   Date _____

Procedure 17-7 | Measuring Color Perception

Name: _____ Date: _____ Time: _____ Grade: _____

Equipment: Ishihara color plate book, disposable gloves

Performance Requirement: Student will perform this skill with ____% accuracy not to exceed _____ minutes. (Instructor will determine the point value for each step, % accuracy, and minutes required.)

Performance Checklist

Point Value	Performance Points Earned	Procedure Steps
		1. Wash your hands. Put on gloves and get the Ishihara color plate book.
		2. Identify the patient by name and explain the procedure. Make sure the patient is seated comfortably in a quiet, well-lighted room.
		3. Hold the first plate in the book about 15–30 inches from the patient. The first plate should be obvious to all patients and serve as an example. Ask the patient if she can see the number formed by the dots on the plate.
		4. Record the patient's results by noting the number of the figure the patient reports for each plate. Write the plate number followed by the patient's response.
		5. Continue showing plates and recording patient responses for plates 1–10. Plate 11 requires the patient to trace a winding bluish-green line between two *X's*. Patients with a color deficit will not be able to trace the line.
		6. Store the color plate book in a closed, protected area to protect the integrity of the colors.
		7. Remove your gloves and wash your hands.

CALCULATION

Total Points Possible: _____

Total Points Earned: _____

Points Earned/Points Possible = _____%

Student completion time (minutes): _____

PASS   FAIL   COMMENTS:

_____

Student's signature _____ Date _____

Instructor's signature _____ Date _____

Procedure 17-8   Assisting with the Pelvic Examination

Name: _____ Date: _____ Time: _____ Grade: _____

Equipment: Patient gown and drape, vaginal speculum, Pap smear collection materials, microscope slides, laboratory requisition, lubricant, disposable gloves, exam light, tissues, basin for used instruments, and biohazard waste container

Performance Requirement: Student will perform this skill with _____% accuracy not to exceed _____ minutes. (Instructor will determine the point value for each step, % accuracy, and minutes required.)

Performance Checklist

Point Value	Performance Points Earned	Procedure Steps
		1. Wash your hands and assemble equipment and supplies. Label microscope slides if used.
		2. Prepare the examination room and the patient.
		3. Greet the patient by name and explain the procedure. Identifying the patient by name prevents errors and may help put her at ease.
		4. Ask the patient to empty her bladder and, if necessary, collect a urine specimen.
		5. Provide the patient with a gown and drape; ask her to disrobe from the waist down unless a breast examination is also being done, and then, have patient disrobe completely.
		6. When the physician is ready assist the patient into lithotomy position with her buttocks at the bottom edge of the table.
		7. Adjust the drape to cover the patient's abdomen and knees, exposing the genitalia. Adjust the light over the genitalia for maximum visibility.
		8. Assist the physician with the examination by handing instruments and supplies as needed.
		9. After putting on examination gloves, hold the glass microscope slides while the physician obtains and makes the smears.
		10. Spray or cover each slide with fixative solution. Hold the slide 4–6 inches from the can and spray lightly once.
		11. When the physician removes the vaginal speculum, have a basin or other container ready to receive it.
		12. Apply about 1–2 inches of lubricant across the physician's two fingers.

Procedure 17-8	Assisting with the Pelvic Examination (*Continued*)

Performance Checklist

Point Value	Performance Points Earned	Procedure Steps
		13. Encourage the patient to relax during the bimanual examination.
		14. After the examination, help the patient slide to the far end of the examination table. Then, remove both feet from the stirrups at the same time.
		15. Offer the patient tissues to remove excess lubricant.
		16. Help her sit up if necessary. Watch the patient for signs of vertigo.
		17. Reinforce any instructions from the physician regarding follow-up appointments.
		18. After the patient leaves, properly care for and dispose of equipment.
		19. Clean the room and remove gloves. Wash your hands.
		20. Document your responsibilities during the procedure, such as routing the specimen to the laboratory and patient education provided.

CALCULATION

Total Points Possible: _____

Total Points Earned: _____

Points Earned/Points Possible = _____%

Student completion time (minutes): _____

PASS   FAIL   COMMENTS:

_____

Student's signature _____ Date _____

Instructor's signature _____ Date _____

18 Assisting with Minor Office Surgery

Chapter Objectives

- Explain the principles and practices of surgical asepsis.
- Describe how to perform a surgical scrub.
- Wrap items for autoclaving.
- Perform sterilization techniques.
- List some of the surgical instruments commonly used in the medical office.
- Summarize how to care for and clean medical instruments.
- Explain how to prepare a treatment room for a surgical procedure, including how to open a sterile surgical pack.
- List possible indicators that a surgical pack has been contaminated.
- Explain how to apply surgical gloves.
- List strategies for maintaining a sterile field.
- Prepare patient for and assist with procedures, treatments, and minor office surgeries.
- Explain how to prepare the patient's skin for minor surgery.
- Identify different methods for wound closure and the necessary supplies.
- Outline the medical assistant's responsibilities in collecting specimens.
- List the responsibilities of the medical assistant following minor surgical procedures.
- Explain how to apply bandages and note the signs of impaired circulation.
- Identify the phases of wound healing and their main characteristics.

CAAHEP & ABHES Competencies

CAAHEP

- Differentiate between medical and surgical asepsis used in ambulatory care setting, indentifying when each is appropriate.
- Document patient care.
- Prepare items for autoclaving.
- Perform sterilization procedures.

ABHES

● Procedure/minor surgery.
● Perform specialty procedures including but not limited to minor surgery, cardiac, respiratory, OB-GYN, neurological, and gastroenterology.

TERMINOLOGY MATCHING

Directions: Match the terms in Column A with the definitions in Column B.

Column A

1. _____ Approximation
2. _____ Autoclave

3. _____ Biopsy
4. _____ Dehiscence

5. _____ Dissect
6. _____ Excise
7. _____ Fenestrated drape

8. _____ Forceps
9. _____ Hemostat
10. _____ Incision

11. _____ Informed consent

12. _____ Medical asepsis
13. _____ Purulent
14. _____ Retractor
15. _____ Sanitizing
16. _____ Scalpel
17. _____ Sterile field

18. _____ Sterilization
19. _____ Surgical asepsis

Column B

a. Cut apart
b. A legal document that explains the course of treatment, including the risks and benefits to the patient
c. A specific area that is considered free of microbes
d. Bringing the edges of the wound as close together as possible to their original position
e. Cut out tissue
f. Stops microbes from spreading from one patient to another
g. The complete elimination or destruction of all microbes, including spores
h. An opening to expose the operative site while covering other areas
i. A device that uses steam heat under high pressure to sterilize objects
j. Used to separate the edges of a wound and to hold open layers of tissue
k. A set of practices designed to keep areas or items free of microorganisms
l. Removal of a tissue sample for diagnostic examination
m. Used for grasping and holding things
n. The separation of wound edges
o. Drainage with a color other than pink
p. Used to grasp and clamp blood vessels
q. Reducing the microorganisms on a surface by using low-level disinfection practices
r. Cutting into tissue
s. Small surgical knife

DEFINING ABBREVIATIONS

Directions: Provide the specific meaning of each of the following abbreviations. Watch your spelling.

20. Bx: _____

_____

21. C&S: _____

_____

22. DSD: _____

_____

23. I&D: _____

_____

MAKING IT RIGHT

Each of the following statements is false. Rewrite the statement to make it a true statement.

24. Sterilization means reducing the microorganisms on a surface by using low-level disinfection practices.

_____

_____

_____

_____

25. The autoclave is the most commonly used piece of equipment for disinfecting instruments.

_____

_____

_____

_____

26. Surgical tape is a special tape placed on the outside of the wrap used to package equipment that is going into the autoclave.

_____

_____

_____

_____

27. Proper sterilization requires three elements, the correct amount of water, 15 minutes, and steam.

_____

_____

_____

_____

28. Surgical packs sterilized on site in an autoclave are considered sterile for 60 days.

_____

_____

_____

_____

29. A sterile transfer forceps is a surgical instrument with slender, straight or curved jaws used to grasp and clamp blood vessels to establish hemostasis.

_____

_____

_____

_____

30. Dissection scissors have a straight top blade with a blunt bottom blade hooked to fit under, lift, and grasp sutures for snipping.

_____

_____

_____

_____

MULTIPLE CHOICE

Directions: Choose the best answer for each question.

31. Which of these is not a reason to use a bandage over a surgical site dressing?

   a. To support an injured body part
   b. To provide additional pressure to control bleeding
   c. To absorb drainage such as blood and pus
   d. To provide protection from contamination
   e. To keep an injured body part immobile during healing

32. Wound drainage that is white, green, or yellow tinged is described as:

   a. serous.
   b. serosanguineous.
   c. sanguineous.
   d. purulent.
   e. copious.

33. Which of these is not a consideration for patients who have an elastic bandage applied?

   a. Increased swelling of the body part
   b. Increased pain of the body part
   c. Pale or cyanotic skin color
   d. Cold skin on the affected extremity
   e. Support and slight immobility of the extremity

34. Medical asepsis is a process that:

   a. stops microbes from spreading from one patient to another.
   b. kills all bacteria and spores.
   c. is a set of practices designed to keep areas or items free of microorganisms.
   d. does not require any personal protective equipment.
   e. only applies to processing surgical instruments.

35. Which of these is not required to perform a surgical hand scrub?

   a. Sterile brush
   b. Alcohol-based hand sanitizer
   c. Sterile towels
   d. Surgical soap in dispenser
   e. Orange stick or nail brush

36. Which of these represents the proper sequence of tasks from start to finish when sterilizing instruments?

    a. Soak instruments in cold water, wrap, and sterilize.
    b. Run water over instruments, wrap in autoclave paper, and sterilize.
    c. Soak instruments in disinfectant solution, wrap, and place in sterilizer.
    d. Disinfect instruments by soaking in solution and place in sterilizer.
    e. Sanitize instruments, allow to dry, and place in sterilizer.

37. The most common method of sterilization in the medical office is:

    a. using disinfecting solutions.
    b. microwaving instruments.
    c. dry heat.
    d. using steam.
    e. gas used in sterilizer.

38. To pull back body tissues to expose other areas during surgery, the physician will use a:

    a. hemostatic forceps.
    b. suture scissor.
    c. retractor.
    d. clamp.
    e. thumb forceps.

39. Which of these is a characteristic of the sterile field?

    a. It is free of microbes.
    b. The sterility of the field is managed by the physician.
    c. Instruments are sterile; however, added items are disinfected.
    d. A sharps container placed on the sterile field is for disposal of sharp items.
    e. A medical assistant wears sterile gloves while setting up the sterile tray.

40. When examining surgical scissors to ensure they are working properly, they should not:

    a. be free of nicks.
    b. have loose box locks.
    c. have tight evenly closing tips.
    d. have no rough areas.
    e. free moving box locks.

41. Which of these is not required on the maintenance records of an autoclave?

    a. Results of the sterilization indicator
    b. The expiration date of the load processed in the autoclave
    c. The name or initials of the autoclave operator
    d. The date and time of each sterilization cycle
    e. Surgical procedures performed each day

42. The primary purpose of sterile transfer forceps is to:

    a. transfer nonsterile instruments to the sterile field.
    b. assist in putting on sterile gloves.
    c. move sterile items on the sterile field.
    d. put unclean instruments in a basin for disinfecting.
    e. hold a vial of medication for the physician.

43. Which of these is a false statement regarding informed consent?

    a. The medical assistant ensures that the patient has signed the informed consent form prior to the surgery.
    b. The patient is required to sign the informed consent form even for minor office procedures.
    c. By signing the informed consent form, the patient agrees that the physician has explained the procedure and possible risks involved.
    d. The medical assistant is responsible to provide a full explanation of any surgical procedure, the risks involved, and answer the patient's questions.
    e. The informed consent form is signed prior to the procedure, not after the procedure.

44. Which of these is a patient question the physician must answer?

    a. Approximately how long will the procedure take?
    b. What are the possible risks if I do not have this procedure?
    c. Do I need to do any preparation before the surgery?
    d. Will my insurance cover the charges?
    e. Is fasting necessary before the procedure?

45. Which of the following items is designed to cover the patient exposing only the operative site?

    a. Gauze pad
    b. Fenestrated drape
    c. Towel
    d. Sterile 4 × 4
    e. Patient gown

46. Which of these is an anesthetic used in the office for minor surgical procedures?

    a. Lidocaine
    b. Benadryl
    c. Penicillin
    d. Cortisone
    e. Betadine

47. The substance added to local anesthetics to cause vasoconstriction is:

    a. Marcaine.
    b. Carbocaine.
    c. mepivacaine.
    d. epinephrine.
    e. bupivacaine.

48. Which of these is not commonly used for closing wounds?

    a. Sutures
    b. Adhesives
    c. Staples
    d. Steri-Strips
    e. Gauze

49. Which of these materials is absorbable suture?

    a. Nylon
    b. Dacron
    c. Polypropylene
    d. Catgut
    e. Stainless steel wire

50. The process where high-frequency electric current is used to excise lesions is:

    a. electrolysis.
    b. electrosurgery.
    c. electrocautery.
    d. cryosurgery.
    e. laser surgery.

51. Which of these types of office surgery does not require sending a tissue specimen to the laboratory?

    a. Cervical biopsy
    b. Excision of a mole
    c. Incision and drainage
    d. Punch biopsy
    e. Excision of a tumor

52. What information is not required on the requisition form that accompanies a tissue specimen?

    a. Patient's insurance company
    b. Patient's name and age
    c. Date the specimen was collected
    d. Type of specimen
    e. Location on the body where the specimen was collected

53. The process used in surgery that causes quick coagulation or clotting of small blood vessels by electric current is:

    a. electrosurgery.
    b. electrodesiccation.
    c. electrocautery.
    d. electrolysis.
    e. fulguration.

54. What information is not included in patient education following minor office surgery?

    a. Postoperative wound care
    b. Scheduling follow-up visits
    c. Signs of infection to watch for
    d. Medication instructions
    e. Insurance billing instructions

55. Sanguineous drainage is:

    a. purulent.
    b. clear.
    c. yellow.
    d. blood tinged.
    e. pus tinged.

56. A 5/8″ tubular gauze bandage is used to:

    a. bandage a finger.
    b. dress an abdominal wound.
    c. cover a wound on the head.
    d. dress a minor surgical site on the neck.
    e. bandage a laceration on the thigh.

57. When bandaging, a figure-8 turn method is used to bandage:

    a. a finger.
    b. the elbow.
    c. the upper arm.
    d. the abdomen.
    e. the large toe.

58. Phase II of wound healing involves:

    a. inflammation.
    b. exudate.
    c. remodeling.
    d. maturation.
    e. granulation.

59. Surgical asepsis is not required when:

    a. handling sterile instruments that break the skin.
    b. changing sterile dressings.
    c. wrapping instruments for sterilization.
    d. assisting with surgical procedures.
    e. performing minor office surgery.

60. What temperature is recommended for proper sterilization of instruments?

    a. 200°F
    b. 212°F
    c. 225°F
    d. 250°F
    e. 275°F

BRIEF EXPLANATIONS

61. Explain the steps in preparing instruments for autoclaving.

    _____
    _____
    _____
    _____

62. Describe the use of each of these instruments.

    Hemostatic forceps: _____

    Suture scissors: _____

    Scalpel: _____

    Retractor: _____

63. Explain the purpose for each of these surgical procedures.

    I&D: _____

    Laceration repair: _____

    Lesion biopsy: _____

64. What is the difference between medical asepsis and surgical asepsis?

_____

_____

_____

_____

65. Explain the difference between sanitization, disinfection, and sterilization.

_____

_____

_____

_____

66. What is the purpose of an informed consent contract? What specific information should be included in the contract?

_____

_____

_____

_____

WHAT DO YOU DO?

67. Read the following scenario and respond to the questions with a short answer.

    Daniel Steen is a new patient who is seeing the physician to have a mole removed from his right forearm. You take his vital signs including temperature, pulse, respiration, and blood pressure. As you review his patient information form, you notice that he is allergic to penicillin and lidocaine. He also indicated on his form that he is taking Coumadin due to a recent deep vein thrombus treated by his former physician.

    a. How would you respond to the patient if he asks if the Coumadin will interfere with his surgical procedure?

    _____

    _____

    _____

    _____

    b. He asks you if there will be sutures put in the surgical site. He also mentions that he will be able to take them out so he will not have to return for a follow-up appointment. How will you respond to these questions and comments?

    _____

    _____

    _____

    _____

c. After the surgical procedure, you begin to put a sterile dressing over the incision site. The patient says you do not have to bother with that since the air is best for healing. How will you explain the need to have the wound covered and kept dry?

_____

_____

_____

_____

PATIENT EDUCATION

68. Write a short narrative script that you can use to provide patient education explaining the things to watch for following a minor office surgery. These should include signs of inflammation and infection.

_____

_____

_____

_____

INTERNET RESEARCH

Visit the Centers for Disease Control and Prevention Web site at www.cdc.gov and research surgical site infections. What information from this site would be good to include in patient education brochures? What statistics are available about the number of postoperative infections?

_____

_____

_____

_____

_____

_____

_____

Procedure 18-1 | Performing a Surgical Scrub

Name: _____ Date: _____ Time: _____ Grade: _____

Equipment: Sink, soap, orange stick or nail brush, and sterile towel

Performance Requirement: Student will perform this skill with ____% accuracy not to exceed _____ minutes. (Instructor will determine the point value for each step, % accuracy, and minutes required.)

Performance Checklist

Point Value	Performance Points Earned	Procedure Steps
		1. Remove rings, watches, or bracelets.
		2. Adjust the water to a comfortable temperature.
		3. Hold your arms at or higher than waist level. Keep your hands higher than your elbows. Otherwise, water may run down from unscrubbed areas of your arms and contaminate your hands. Do not let your clothing touch the sink.
		4. Use an orange stick or nail brush to clean under each nail. Then, discard the orange stick taking care not to touch the insides of the sink or the faucet.
		5. Apply surgical soap and wash your hands thoroughly. Use a firm circular motion. Hold your fingers up and rub each side of each finger, between the fingers, and the back and front of each hand. This process should take about 5 minutes for each hand.
		6. Keeping your hands higher than your elbows, wash your wrists and forearms thoroughly with soap. Rinse your arms and hands under running water without touching the sides of the sink or faucet.
		7. Using more surgical soap and a sterile brush, scrub all the surfaces you just washed. Follow a systematic approach. Begin with your fingers and then scrub your hands and finally your arms.
		8. Discard the sterile brush and rinse your hands and arms by passing them through the running water in one direction—from the hand to the elbow.
		9. Turn off the faucet using the foot or arm mechanism.
		10. Dry your hands using a sterile towel. Use one end of the towel to dry one hand, then the arm, then the forearm. Use the other clean end of the towel to dry the other hand, arm, and forearm.
		11. Discard the scrub brush and used towel.

(Continued)

Procedure 18-1   Performing a Surgical Scrub (*Continued*)

CALCULATION

Total Points Possible: _____

Total Points Earned: _____

Points Earned/Points Possible = _____%

Student completion time (minutes): _____

PASS   FAIL   COMMENTS:

_____

Student's signature _____   Date _____

Instructor's signature _____   Date _____

Procedure 18-2   Applying Sterile Gloves

Name: _____   Date: _____   Time: _____   Grade: _____

Equipment: Sterile gloves

Performance Requirement: Student will perform this skill with ____% accuracy not to exceed _____ minutes.
(Instructor will determine the point value for each step, % accuracy, and minutes required.)

Performance Checklist

Point Value	Performance Points Earned	Procedure Steps
		1. Remove any rings or other jewelry.
		2. Wash your hands before applying gloves.
		3. Place the glove package on a clean, dry, flat surface with the cuffed end of the glove facing you.
		4. Pull the outer wrapping apart to expose the sterile, inner wrap.
		5. With the cuffs toward you, fold back the inner wrap to expose the gloves.
		6. Grasp the edges of the outer paper, and open the package out to its fullest.
		7. Using your nondominant hand, pick up the dominant hand glove by grasping the folded edge of the cuff. Lift it up and away from the paper to avoid brushing an unsterile surface.
		8. Curl your fingers and thumb together and insert them into the glove. Straighten your fingers and pull the glove on with your nondominant hand still grasping the cuff.
		9. Unfold the cuff by pinching the inside surface that will be against your wrist and pulling it toward your wrist. Touch only the unsterile portions of the glove with your hands.
		10. Place the fingers of your gloved hand under the cuff of the remaining glove. Lift the glove up and away from the wrapper to prevent it from touching an unsterile surface.
		11. Slide your ungloved hand carefully into the glove with your fingers and thumb curled together.
		12. Straighten your fingers and pull the glove up and over your wrist by carefully unfolding the glove.
		13. Settle the gloves comfortably onto your fingers by lacing your fingers together and adjusting the tension over your hands. The gloves should fit snugly without wrinkles or areas that bind the fingers.

(Continued)

| Procedure 18-2 | Applying Sterile Gloves (*Continued*) |

CALCULATION

Total Points Possible: _____

Total Points Earned: _____

Points Earned/Points Possible = _____%

Student completion time (minutes): _____

PASS   FAIL   COMMENTS:

_____

Student's signature _____   Date _____

Instructor's signature _____   Date _____

Procedure 18-3	Wrapping Instruments for Sterilization in an Autoclave

Name: _____ Date: _____ Time: _____ Grade: _____

Equipment: Autoclave wrapping material, autoclave tape, sterilization indicators, and black or blue ink pen

Performance Requirement: Student will perform this skill with ____% accuracy not to exceed _____ minutes. (Instructor will determine the point value for each step, % accuracy, and minutes required.)

Performance Checklist

Point Value	Performance Points Earned	Procedure Steps
		1. Wash your hands and put on nonsterile gloves. Gather the instruments to be sterilized and the necessary supplies.
		2. Check the instruments being wrapped to be sure they have been sanitized, disinfected, and dry. Check that they are in working order.
		3. Tear off one piece of autoclave tape. Write the date, your initials, and the contents of the pack or the name of the instrument in the pack.
		4. Lay the wrapping material diagonally on a flat, clean, dry surface. Place the instrument(s) in the center of the wrapping material.
		5. Ensure ratchets or handles are open to allow steam to circulate.
		6. Place sterilization indicator in middle of pack.
		7. Fold the flap at the bottom of the diagonal wrap up. Fold back the corner to make a tab.
		8. Fold the left corner of the wrap in to the center. Fold back the corner to make a tab. Do the same for the right corner of the wrap.
		9. Fold the top corner down, tucking the tab under the material.
		10. Secure the wrapped instrument package with the labeled autoclave tape.
		11. Remove gloves and wash hands.

(Continued)

Procedure 18-3 | Wrapping Instruments for Sterilization in an Autoclave (*Continued*)

CALCULATION

Total Points Possible: _____

Total Points Earned: _____

Points Earned/Points Possible = _____%

Student completion time (minutes): _____

PASS   FAIL   COMMENTS:

_____

Student's signature _____   Date _____

Instructor's signature_____   Date _____

Procedure 18-4 Operating an Autoclave

Name: _____ Date: _____ Time: _____ Grade: _____

Equipment: Autoclave, wrapped packs, and distilled water

Performance Requirement: Student will perform this skill with ____% accuracy not to exceed _____ minutes. (Instructor will determine the point value for each step, % accuracy, and minutes required.)

Performance Checklist

Point Value	Performance Points Earned	Procedure Steps
		1. Gather items for sterilization.
		2. Check the water level in the autoclave reservoir. Add more distilled water if necessary.
		3. Add water to the internal chamber of the autoclave. Make sure the water level is at the fill line.
		4. Load the autoclave following loading guidelines.
		5. Follow manufacturer's instructions for closing and operating the machine.
		6. When the load has cooled, remove the items. Check the sterilization indicator, if one was included in the autoclave or on each pack.
		7. Store the items in a clean, dry, dust-free area for 30 days.
		8. Clean the autoclave according to the manufacturer's directions.

CALCULATION

Total Points Possible: _____

Total Points Earned: _____

Points Earned/Points Possible = _____%

Student completion time (minutes): _____

PASS   FAIL   COMMENTS:

_____

Student's signature _____ Date _____

Instructor's signature _____ Date _____

Procedure 18-5 | Performing Chemical Sterilization

Name: _____ Date: _____ Time: _____ Grade: _____

Equipment: Sterilization chemical, safety data sheet, PPE, heavy-duty utility gloves, stainless steel or glass container with airtight cover, sterile water, sterile basin, sterile transfer forceps, sterile towels, and items for sterilization

Performance Requirement: Student will perform this skill with ____% accuracy not to exceed _____ minutes. (Instructor will determine the point value for each step, % accuracy, and minutes required.)

Performance Checklist

Point Value	Performance Points Earned	Procedure Steps
		1. Put on disposable gloves, goggles, and other PPE to protect your eyes, clothing, and exposed skin from possible harmful chemicals.
		2. Scrub and sanitize the items to be sterilized to remove debris and body fluids.
		3. Rinse and dry the items. They must be dry when placed in the chemical sterilization solution in order to avoid diluting the solution.
		4. Check the expiration date on the container of the sterilization chemical. If the chemical is used past its expiration date, it may not be as effective.
		5. Read the manufacturer's instructions on the container of the sterilization chemical, and review the SDS for the chemical used.
		6. Put on the heavy-duty utility gloves over the disposable PPE gloves.
		7. Mix or prepare the solution according to the manufacturer's directions on the label.
		8. Pour the solution into a glass or stainless steel container with an airtight lid. Cover the solution in order to avoid loss of potency through evaporation or injury from splashes or inhalation of fumes.
		9. Carefully place the dry sanitized items into the container in order to avoid splashing, completely covering by the solution. Replace the container's airtight lid.
		10. Label the lid with the name of the chemical, the date and time, and the length of time required for sterilization.
		11. Leave the items in the solution for the required time. Do not open the container or add more items during this time.
		12. After the recommended processing time has expired, open the container and remove each item from the solution using sterile transfer forceps.

Procedure 18-5 Performing Chemical Sterilization (*Continued*)

Performance Checklist

Point Value	Performance Points Earned	Procedure Steps
		13. With the sterile forceps, hold the item over a sterile basin and pour large amounts of sterile water over and through it. This removes all traces of the chemical solution from the item.
		14. Continue to hold the item over the sterile basin for a moment to allow the excess water to drain off. Then, place the item on a sterile towel.
		15. After all the items have been removed from the container, rinsed, and transferred onto sterile towels, dry them with another sterile towel. Take care to avoid touching the instruments or the side of the towel while drying them.
		16. Use the sterile transfer forceps to place the items in storage for future use according to the office procedures.

CALCULATION

Total Points Possible: _____

Total Points Earned: _____

Points Earned/Points Possible = _____ %

Student completion time (minutes): _____

PASS   FAIL   COMMENTS:

_____

Student's signature _____ Date _____

Instructor's signature _____ Date _____

Procedure 18-6   Opening Sterile Packs

Name: _____ Date: _____ Time: _____ Grade: _____

Equipment: Sterile pack

Performance Requirement: Student will perform this skill with _____% accuracy not to exceed _____ minutes. (Instructor will determine the point value for each step, % accuracy, and minutes required.)

Performance Checklist

Point Value	Performance Points Earned	Procedure Steps
		1. Verify the procedure scheduled to be performed and remove the appropriate surgical pack (tray or item) from the storage area.
		2. Check the label for the contents and expiration date.
		3. Check the package for tears, stains, and moisture, which would suggest contamination.
		4. Place the package, with the label facing up, on a clean, dry, flat surface, such as a Mayo or surgical stand.
		5. Wash your hands. Carefully remove the sealing tape. Take care not to tear the wrapper.
		6. Loosen the first flap of the folded wrapper by pulling it up, out, and away from you. Let it fall over the far side of the table or stand. Then, you will not need to reach across the sterile field again.
		7. Open the side flaps in a similar manner to minimize your movements over the sterile field. Use your left hand for the left flap and your right hand for the right flap. Touch only the outer surface. Do not touch the sterile inner surface.
		8. Grasp the outer surface of the remaining flap. Pull it down and toward you. The outer surface of the wrapper should now be against the surgical stand. The sterile inside of the wrapper forms the sterile field.
		9. Some packages have a second inside wrapper. Repeat steps 6–8 to open the second wrapper. It also will provide a sterile field.
		10. If you need to leave the area after opening the sterile field, cover the tray and its contents with a sterile drape.

Procedure 18-6 | Opening Sterile Packs (*Continued*)

CALCULATION

Total Points Possible: _____

Total Points Earned: _____

Points Earned/Points Possible = _____%

Student completion time (minutes): _____

PASS   FAIL   COMMENTS:

_____

Student's signature _____   Date _____

Instructor's signature _____   Date _____

Procedure 18-7 | Using Sterile Transfer Forceps

Name: _____ Date: _____ Time: _____ Grade: _____

Equipment: Sterile transfer forceps in solution and various items to transfer to sterile field

Performance Requirement: Student will perform this skill with ____% accuracy not to exceed _____ minutes. (Instructor will determine the point value for each step, % accuracy, and minutes required.)

Performance Checklist

Point Value	Performance Points Earned	Procedure Steps
		1. Slowly lift the forceps straight up and out of the container with solution. Do not touch the outside of the container or the inside of the container above the level of the solution.
		2. Hold the forceps with the tips down at all times. This prevents contamination by preventing the solution from running up toward the unsterile handles and then down to the grasping blades and tips. Keep the forceps above waist level to avoid accidental or unnoticed contamination.
		3. Use the forceps to pick up items to transfer onto the sterile field. Drop the items carefully onto the field.
		4. When finished moving items, carefully place the forceps back into the sterilization solution.

CALCULATION

Total Points Possible: _____

Total Points Earned: _____

Points Earned/Points Possible = _____%

Student completion time (minutes): _____

PASS   FAIL   COMMENTS:

_____

Student's signature _____ Date _____

Instructor's signature _____ Date _____

Procedure 18-8 | Adding Sterile Solution

Name: _____ Date: _____ Time: _____ Grade: _____

Equipment: Sterile bowl or cup on a sterile field, sterile transfer forceps, and solution

Performance Requirement: Student will perform this skill with _____% accuracy not to exceed _____ minutes. (Instructor will determine the point value for each step, % accuracy, and minutes required.)

Performance Checklist

Point Value	Performance Points Earned	Procedure Steps
		1. Place a sterile bowl or cup on the sterile field using sterile transfer forceps.
		2. Identify the correct solution by carefully reading the label. Check the label three times to prevent errors.
		3. Check the expiration date on the solution label.
		4. If adding medication, such as lidocaine, to the solution, show the medication label to the physician.
		5. Remove the cap or stopper on the bottle. Hold the cap with your fingertips, with the opening facing down to prevent contamination.
		6. If you must put the cap down, place it on a side table (not the sterile field) with the open end up.
		7. Grasp the container with the label against the palm of your hand.
		8. Pour a small amount of the solution into a separate container or waste receptacle. The lip of the bottle is considered contaminated. Pouring off this small amount cleanses the lip.
		9. Without reaching across the sterile field, carefully and slowly pour the desired amount of solution into the sterile container.
		10. After pouring the solution, recheck the label for the contents and expiration date. Replace the cap carefully, without touching the bottle rim with any unsterile surface of the cap.
		11. Return the solution to its proper storage area or discard the container after checking the label again.

(Continued)

Procedure 18-8 | Adding Sterile Solution (*Continued*)

CALCULATION

Total Points Possible: _____

Total Points Earned: _____

Points Earned/Points Possible = _____%

Student completion time (minutes): _____

PASS   FAIL   COMMENTS:

_____

Student's signature _____   Date _____

Instructor's signature_____   Date _____

Procedure 18-9 | Performing Hair Removal and Skin Preparation

Name: _____ Date: _____ Time: _____ Grade: _____

Equipment: Nonsterile gloves; shaving cream, lotion, or soap; a new disposable razor; gauze or cotton balls; warm water; antiseptic solution; and sponge forceps

Performance Requirement: Student will perform this skill with _____% accuracy not to exceed _____ minutes. (Instructor will determine the point value for each step, % accuracy, and minutes required.)

Performance Checklist

Point Value	Performance Points Earned	Procedure Steps
		1. Wash your hands and gather equipment and supplies.
		2. Greet the patient by name and explain the procedure. Answer any questions the patient may have.
		3. Put on gloves.
		4. Prepare the patient's skin. If shaving is required apply shaving cream or soapy lather to the area to reduce friction. Pull the skin taut and shave by pulling the razor across the skin in the direction of hair growth.
		5. Thoroughly dry the area by patting with gauze square.
		6. If shaving is not necessary, wash and rinse the patient's skin with soap and water. Dry the skin thoroughly.
		7. Apply antiseptic solution of the physician's choice to the skin surrounding the operative area. Use sterile gauze sponges or sterile cotton balls to apply the solution, or use antiseptic wipes. Hold the gauze or cotton ball in sterile sponge forceps.
		8. Wipe the skin in circular motions, beginning at the operative site and working outward. Discard each sponge after a complete sweep to prevent contamination.
		9. Holding dry sterile sponges in the sponge forceps, thoroughly pat the area dry, or in some instances, allow the area to air dry.
		10. Tell the patient not to touch or cover the prepared area to avoid contaminating the operative site.
		11. Inform the physician that the patient is ready for the procedure. Drape the prepared area with a sterile drape if the physician is delayed for more than 10 or 15 minutes.

(Continued)

Procedure 18-9 | Performing Hair Removal and Skin Preparation (*Continued*)

CALCULATION

Total Points Possible: _____

Total Points Earned: _____

Points Earned/Points Possible = _____%

Student completion time (minutes): _____

PASS   FAIL   COMMENTS:

_____

Student's signature _____   Date _____

Instructor's signature _____   Date _____

Procedure 18-10   Assisting with Excisional Surgery

Name: _____ Date: _____ Time: _____ Grade: _____

Equipment: Sterile field with basin for solutions, gauze sponges and cotton balls, antiseptic solution, a sterile drape, sterile syringes and needles for local anesthetic, dissecting scissors, a disposable scalpel, a blade of the physician's choice, mosquito forceps, tissue forceps, a needle holder, and a suture and needle of the physician's choice. At the side, place sterile gloves, local anesthetic, antiseptic wipes, adhesive tape, sterile dressings, and a specimen container with a completed laboratory request form.

Performance Requirement: Student will perform this skill with _____% accuracy not to exceed _____ minutes. (Instructor will determine the point value for each step, % accuracy, and minutes required.)

Performance Checklist

Point Value	Performance Points Earned	Procedure Steps
		1. Wash your hands and gather equipment and supplies.
		2. Greet the patient by name and explain the procedure. Answer any questions the patient may have.
		3. Set up a sterile field on a surgical stand with the at-the-side supplies and equipment close at hand. Cover the field with a sterile drape until the physician arrives.
		4. Position the patient appropriately to expose the operative site.
		5. Put on sterile gloves or use sterile transfer forceps and cleanse the patient's skin. When finished, remove your gloves and wash your hands.
		6. If the physician asks you, assist during the procedure. You may need to add supplies, watch for opportunities to assist the physician, and comfort the patient. You do not need to wear sterile gloves unless handling sterile instruments or supplies.
		7. If the lesion is sent to pathology for analysis, you will need to assist in specimen collection. Follow standard precautions and wear examination gloves when handling specimens. Have the container ready to receive the specimen.
		8. At the end of the procedure, wash your hands and dress the wound using sterile technique. Cover the wound to protect the incision from contamination.
		9. Thank the patient and provide instructions for postoperative care, including dressing changes, postoperative medications, and follow-up visits.
		10. Wearing gloves, clean the treatment room and prepare it for the next patient. Follow standard precautions.
		11. Record the procedure. Documentation includes postoperative vital signs, care of the wound, instructions on postoperative care, and processing any specimens.

(Continued)

Procedure 18-10   **Assisting with Excisional Surgery (*Continued*)**

CALCULATION

Total Points Possible: _____

Total Points Earned: _____

Points Earned/Points Possible = _____%

Student completion time (minutes): _____

PASS   FAIL   COMMENTS:

_____

Student's signature _____   Date _____

Instructor's signature _____   Date _____

Procedure 18-11 | Assisting with Colposcopy and Cervical Biopsy

Name: _____ Date: _____ Time: _____ Grade: _____

Equipment: Sterile gloves, a gown and drape, a vaginal speculum, a colposcope, a specimen container with preservative (10% formalin), sterile cotton-tipped applicators, sterile normal saline solution, sterile 3% acetic acid, sterile povidone–iodine (Betadine), silver nitrate sticks or ferric subsulfate (Monsel solution), sterile biopsy forceps or punch biopsy instrument, a sterile uterine curette, sterile uterine dressing forceps, sterile 4 × 4 gauze, a sterile towel, a sterile endocervical curette, a sterile uterine tenaculum, a sanitary napkin, examination gloves, an examination light, tissues, and biohazard container.

Performance Requirement: Student will perform this skill with _____% accuracy not to exceed _____ minutes. (Instructor will determine the point value for each step, % accuracy, and minutes required.)

Performance Checklist

Point Value	Performance Points Earned	Procedure Steps
		1. Label a specimen container with the patient's name and date.
		2. Wash your hands and gather equipment and supplies.
		3. Check the light on the colposcope to make sure it's functioning properly.
		4. Set up the sterile field using sterile technique. Items placed on the sterile field include the sterile cotton-tipped applicators and sterile containers for the solutions.
		5. Pour sterile normal saline and acetic acid into their sterile containers. Cover the field with a drape to maintain sterility as you prepare the patient.
		6. Greet the patient by name and explain the procedure, answering any last-minute questions from the patient.
		7. When the physician is ready, assist the patient into the dorsal lithotomy position. If you are going to be assisting the physician from the sterile field, put on sterile gloves after you position the patient.
		8. Hand the physician the applicator immersed in normal saline followed by the applicator immersed in acetic acid. Acetic acid swabbed on the area improves visualization of abnormal tissue.
		9. Hand the physician the applicator with the antiseptic solution (Betadine).
		10. If you didn't apply sterile gloves to assist the physician, apply clean examination gloves. Receive the biopsy specimen into the container of 10% formalin preservative.

(Continued)

Procedure 18-11 | Assisting with Colposcopy and Cervical Biopsy (*Continued*)

Performance Checklist

Point Value	Performance Points Earned	Procedure Steps
		11. If necessary, provide the physician with Monsel solution or silver nitrate sticks to stop any bleeding.
		12. When the physician is finished, remove your gloves and wash your hands. Assist the patient from the stirrups and into a sitting position.
		13. Explain to the patient that a small amount of bleeding may occur. Have a sanitary napkin available.
		14. Ask the patient to get dressed and assist as needed. Allow the patient privacy for dressing.
		15. Reinforce any instructions from the physician regarding follow-up appointments. Tell the patient how to obtain the biopsy findings.
		16. Wearing gloves, properly care for or dispose of equipment and clean the examination room. Remove your gloves and wash your hands.
		17. Document the procedure, including routing the specimen and patient education.

CALCULATION

Total Points Possible: _____

Total Points Earned: _____

Points Earned/Points Possible = _____%

Student completion time (minutes): _____

PASS   FAIL   COMMENTS:

_____

Student's signature _____ Date _____

Instructor's signature _____ Date _____

Procedure 18-12 | Assisting with Incision and Drainage

Name: _____ Date: _____ Time: _____ Grade: _____

Equipment: On sterile field, a basin for solutions, gauze sponges and cotton balls, antiseptic solution, a sterile drape, sterile syringes and sterile needles for local anesthetic, a commercial incision and drainage sterile setup *or* scalpel, dissecting scissors, hemostats, tissue forceps, sterile 4 × 4 gauze sponges, and a probe. At the side, place sterile gloves, local anesthetic, antiseptic wipes, adhesive tape, sterile dressings, packing gauze, and a culture tube if the wound may be cultured.

Performance Requirement: Student will perform this skill with _____% accuracy not to exceed _____ minutes. (Instructor will determine the point value for each step, % accuracy, and minutes required.)

Performance Checklist

Point Value	Performance Points Earned	Procedure Steps
		1. Wash your hands and gather the equipment.
		2. Greet the patient by name and explain the procedure. Answer any questions the patient may have.
		3. Set up a sterile field on a surgical stand with the at-the-side supplies and equipment. Cover the field with a sterile drape until the physician arrives.
		4. Position the patient appropriately to expose the operative site.
		5. Put on sterile gloves or use sterile transfer forceps and cleanse the patient's skin. When finished, remove your gloves and wash your hands.
		6. If the physician asks you, assist during the procedure. You may need to add supplies, watch for opportunities to assist the physician, and comfort the patient. You do not need to wear sterile gloves unless handling sterile instruments or supplies.
		7. Label the specimen container and prepare a laboratory request if a culture and sensitivity has been ordered.
		8. At the end of the procedure, wash your hands and dress the wound using sterile technique. Cover the wound to protect the incision from contamination.
		9. Thank the patient and provide instructions for postoperative care, including dressing changes, postoperative medications, and follow-up visits.
		10. Wearing gloves, clean the treatment room and prepare it for the next patient. Follow standard precautions.
		11. Record the procedure. Documentation includes postoperative vital signs, care of the wound, instructions on postoperative care, and processing any specimens.

(Continued)

Procedure 18-12 | **Assisting with Incision and Drainage** (*Continued*)

CALCULATION

Total Points Possible: _____

Total Points Earned: _____

Points Earned/Points Possible = _____%

Student completion time (minutes): _____

PASS   FAIL   COMMENTS:

_____

Student's signature _____   Date _____

Instructor's signature_____   Date _____

Procedure 18-13 | Applying a Sterile Dressing

Name: _____ Date: _____ Time: _____ Grade: _____

Equipment: Sterile gloves, sterile gauze dressings, scissors, bandage tape, and any medication to be applied to the dressing, according to the physician's orders.

Performance Requirement: Student will perform this skill with ____% accuracy not to exceed _____ minutes. (Instructor will determine the point value for each step, % accuracy, and minutes required.)

Performance Checklist

Point Value	Performance Points Earned	Procedure Steps
		1. Wash your hands and gather the equipment and supplies.
		2. Greet the patient by name and ask about any tape allergies. Some patients are sensitive to certain tape adhesives. Hypoallergenic tape should be available.
		3. Depending on the size of the dressing, cut or tear lengths of tape to secure the dressing. Set the tape strips aside in a convenient place, such as affixing the end of each piece to a nearby countertop for easy removal.
		4. Explain the procedure and instruct the patient to remain still. The patient should avoid talking, sneezing, or coughing until the procedure is complete.
		5. Open the dressing pack to create a sterile field, leaving the sterile dressing on the inside of the opened package. Observe the principles of sterile asepsis.
		6. Use sterile technique to prevent wound contamination. Put on sterile gloves if you will not be using sterile transfer forceps to apply the dressing.
		7. If a topical medication is needed, apply it to the sterile dressing that will cover the wound directly. Take care not to touch the medication bottle or tube to the dressing. Allow the medication to free fall onto the sterile dressing.
		8. Using sterile technique, apply the number of dressings necessary to cover and protect the wound. Apply the previously cut lengths of tape over the dressing to secure it.
		9. When the wound is completely covered, you may remove your gloves.
		10. Apply a bandage if necessary to hold the dressing in place, add support, or immobilize the area.

(Continued)

Procedure 18-13 Applying a Sterile Dressing (*Continued*)

Performance Checklist

Point Value	Performance Points Earned	Procedure Steps
		11. If the patient needs to change dressings at home, instruct the patient on how to do so. Instruct the patient about wound care and signs of infection.
		12. Return reusable supplies to their storage areas. Properly discard contaminated supplies or waste.
		13. Record the procedure in the patient's chart.

CALCULATION

Total Points Possible: _____

Total Points Earned: _____

Points Earned/Points Possible = _____%

Student completion time (minutes): _____

PASS   FAIL   COMMENTS:

_____

Student's signature _____ Date _____

Instructor's signature_____ Date _____

Procedure 18-14 | Changing an Existing Dressing

Name: _____ Date: _____ Time: _____ Grade: _____

Equipment: Sterile gloves, nonsterile gloves, sterile dressing, prepackaged skin antiseptic swabs or sterile antiseptic solution in a sterile basin and sterile cotton balls or gauze, tape, and biohazard waste containers

Performance Requirement: Student will perform this skill with _____% accuracy not to exceed _____ minutes. (Instructor will determine the point value for each step, % accuracy, and minutes required.)

Performance Checklist

Point Value	Performance Points Earned	Procedure Steps
		1. Wash your hands and gather the equipment and supplies.
		2. Greet the patient by name and explain the procedure. Answer any questions the patient may have.
		3. Prepare a sterile field, including opening sterile dressings.
		4. If using a sterile container and solution, open the package containing the sterile basin. Use the inside of the wrapper as the sterile field for the basin.
		5. Flip the sterile gauze or cotton balls into the basin. Pour in the appropriate amount of antiseptic solution.
		6. If using prepackaged antiseptic swabs, carefully open an adequate number for the size of the wound. Set them aside using sterile technique to avoid contamination.
		7. Instruct the patient not to talk, cough, sneeze, laugh, or move during the procedure in order to prevent contamination of the sterile field.
		8. Wearing clean gloves, carefully remove the tape from the wound by pulling it toward the wound. Pulling away from the direction of the wound may pull the healing edges of the wound apart.
		9. Remove the old dressing. Discard the soiled dressing in a biohazard waste container.
		10. Before cleaning, inspect the wound for degree of healing, amount and type of drainage, and appearance of wound edges.
		11. Remove and discard your gloves using medical aseptic practices.
		12. Put on sterile gloves. Clean the wound with the antiseptic solution ordered by the physician.
		13. Remove your gloves and wash your hands. Change the dressing using the procedure for sterile dressing application.
		14. Record the procedure.

(Continued)

| Procedure 18-14 | Changing an Existing Dressing (*Continued*) |

CALCULATION

Total Points Possible: _____

Total Points Earned: _____

Points Earned/Points Possible = _____%

Student completion time (minutes): _____

PASS   FAIL   COMMENTS:

_____

Student's signature _____   Date _____

Instructor's signature_____   Date _____

Procedure 18-15 Removing Sutures

Name: _____ Date: _____ Time: _____ Grade: _____

Equipment: Skin antiseptic, sterile gloves, prepackaged suture removal kit *or* thumb forceps, suture scissors, and gauze.

Performance Requirement: Student will perform this skill with ____% accuracy not to exceed _____ minutes. (Instructor will determine the point value for each step, % accuracy, and minutes required.)

Performance Checklist

Point Value	Performance Points Earned	Procedure Steps
		1. Wash your hands and gather the equipment and supplies.
		2. Apply clean examination gloves.
		3. Check the chart before you begin the procedure to see how many sutures or staples were applied.
		4. Greet the patient by name and explain the procedure. Answer any questions the patient may have.
		5. If dressings are still in place, remove them and dispose of them in biohazard waste containers. Remove your gloves and wash your hands.
		6. Wearing clean examination gloves, cleanse the wound with antiseptic, such as Betadine. Use new antiseptic gauze for each swipe down the wound.
		7. Open the suture removal kit using sterile asepsis technique or set up a sterile field.
		8. Put on sterile gloves.
		9. With the thumb forceps, grasp the end of the suture knot closest to the skin. Lift it slightly and gently up from the skin.
		10. Cut the suture below the knot as close to the skin as possible.
		11. Use the thumb forceps to pull the suture out of the skin with a smooth, continuous motion.
		12. Place the suture on the gauze sponge. Repeat the procedure for each suture. Count the number removed.
		13. Clean the site with an antiseptic solution. Cover it with a sterile dressing if the physician has directed you to do so.
		14. Thank the patient and properly dispose of equipment and supplies. Clean the treatment area, remove your gloves, and wash your hands.
		15. Record the procedure. Documentation must include the time, location of sutures, number removed, and the condition of the wound.

(Continued)

| Procedure 18-15 | Removing Sutures (*Continued*) |

CALCULATION

Total Points Possible: _____

Total Points Earned: _____

Points Earned/Points Possible = _____%

Student completion time (minutes): _____

PASS   FAIL   COMMENTS:

_____

Student's signature _____   Date _____

Instructor's signature _____   Date _____

Procedure 18-16 | Removing Staples

Name: _____ Date: _____ Time: _____ Grade: _____

Equipment: Antiseptic solution or wipes, examination gloves, sterile gloves, sponge forceps, gauze squares, and prepackaged sterile staple removal instrument

Performance Requirement: Student will perform this skill with ____% accuracy not to exceed _____ minutes. (Instructor will determine the point value for each step, % accuracy, and minutes required.)

Performance Checklist

Point Value	Performance Points Earned	Procedure Steps
		1. Wash your hands and gather the equipment and supplies.
		2. Greet the patient by name and explain the procedure. Answer any questions the patient may have.
		3. If the dressing is still in place, put on clean examination gloves and remove it. Dispose of it in a biohazard waste container. Remove your gloves and wash your hands.
		4. Clean the wound with antiseptic. Pat dry with sterile gauze sponges.
		5. Put on sterile gloves.
		6. Gently slide the end of the staple remover under each staple to be removed. Press the handles together to lift the ends of the staples out of the skin.
		7. Place each staple on a gauze square as it is removed.
		8. When all the staples have been removed, gently clean the site with antiseptic solution.
		9. Pat dry and dress the site if the physician has ordered you to do so. The wound may be healed well enough to be left uncovered.
		10. Thank the patient and properly dispose of equipment and supplies. Clean the treatment area, remove your gloves, and wash your hands.
		11. Record the procedure. Documentation must include the time, location of staples, number removed, and the condition of the wound.

(Continued)

Procedure 18-16 Removing Staples (*Continued*)

CALCULATION

Total Points Possible: _____

Total Points Earned: _____

Points Earned/Points Possible = _____%

Student completion time (minutes): _____

PASS   FAIL   COMMENTS:

_____

Student's signature _____ Date _____

Instructor's signature _____ Date _____

19 Pharmacology and Drug Administration

Chapter Objectives

- List the different ways patients receive medications from the physician.
- Identify the three different names associated with most medications.
- Describe the Schedule of Controlled Substances and provide an example of each.
- Explain how to monitor the office inventory of controlled substances.
- Maintain medication records.
- Describe how to prepare a written prescription as directed by a physician.
- Define what is meant by local effect and systemic effect for drug action.
- Discuss the four general processes involved in pharmacokinetics.
- Describe the main factors that influence a drug's effect on the body.
- List resources for finding out more about medications.
- List safety guidelines to follow when administering medications.
- Identify three measuring systems used for medications.
- Explain how to calculate adult and child medication doses.
- Apply pharmacology principles to prepare and administer oral and parenteral medications, excluding IV administration.
- List the different types of injections, their appropriate needle lengths, and their sites of administration.
- Explain what to do in the case of a medication error.
- List the seven rights to check for reducing the risk of medication errors.

CAAHEP & ABHES Competencies

CAAHEP

- Prepare proper dosages of medication for administration.
- Verify ordered doses/dosages prior to administration.
- Select proper sites for administering parenteral medication.
- Administer oral medications.
- Administer parenteral (excluding IV) medications.

- Demonstrate knowledge of basic math computations.
- Apply mathematical computations to solve equations.
- Identify measurement systems.
- Define basic units of measurement in metric, apothecary, and household systems.
- Convert among measurement systems.
- Identify both abbreviations and symbols used in calculating medication dosages.

ABHES

- Identify drug classification, usual dose, side effects, and contraindications of the top most commonly used medications.
- Demonstrate accurate occupational math and metric conversions for proper medication administration.
- Identify parts of prescriptions.
- Identify appropriate abbreviations that are accepted in prescription writing.
- Comply with legal aspects of creating prescriptions, including federal and state laws.
- Properly utilize Physician's Desk Reference (PDR), drug handbook, and other drug references to identify a drug's classification, usual dosage, usual side effects, and contraindications.

TERMINOLOGY MATCHING

Directions: Match the terms in Column A with the definitions in Column B.

Column A

1. _____ Antagonism
2. _____ Allergy
3. _____ Anaphylaxis
4. _____ Ampule
5. _____ Diluent

6. _____ Generic
7. _____ Induration
8. _____ Infiltration
9. _____ Inhalation
10. _____ Inscription
11. _____ Instillation
12. _____ Interaction

13. _____ Parenteral
14. _____ Pharmacokinetic
15. _____ Potentiation
16. _____ Sublingual
17. _____ Subscription

18. _____ Synergism
19. _____ Vial

20. _____ Transdermal
21. _____ Wheal

Column B

a. Located below or beside the symbol Rx, the name of the medication, the desired form, and the strength
b. Small glass containers that must be broken at the neck
c. Tells the pharmacist how much of the drug to dispense
d. An effect in which one drug makes the other less effective
e. How the drugs move through the body after swallowed or injected
f. Through the skin
g. Diluting agent, usually sterile water or saline
h. Administration of a liquid drop by drop
i. Means that two drugs work together.
j. A glass or plastic container that is sealed at the top by a stopper
k. Excessive reaction to a substance
l. The name assigned to the drug during research and development. It refers to the chemical ingredients that make up the drug
m. Severe allergic reaction
n. A small bubble raised in the skin
o. Through the lungs
p. Any route other than the enteral ones
q. Occurs when one drug extends or multiplies the effect of another drug
r. Under the tongue
s. The effect or action that occurs between drugs and the human body
t. IV fluid infuses into tissues surrounding the vein
u. Hard, raised area over an intradermal injection site

DEFINING ABBREVIATIONS

Directions: Provide the specific meaning of each of the following abbreviations. Watch your spelling.

22. BNDD: _____

_____

23. BSA: _____

_____

24. DEA: _____

_____

25. FDA: _____

_____

26. ID: _____

_____

27. IM: _____

_____

28. IV: _____

_____

29. NKA: _____

_____

30. NPO: _____

_____

31. OTC: _____

_____

32. PDR: _____

_____

33. PO: _____

_____

34. Rx: _____

_____

35. SC: _____

_____

36. SQ: _____

_____

37. STAT: _____

_____

38. TB: _____

_____

MAKING IT RIGHT

Each of the following statements is false. Rewrite the statement to make it a true statement.

39. To administer a drug means a written order is given to the patient and taken to a pharmacist to be filled.

_____

_____

_____

_____

40. Prescription-only medications are usually available in pharmacies and supermarkets without any restrictions.

_____

_____

_____

_____

41. Analgesic medications neutralize or reduce stomach acidity.

_____

_____

_____

_____

42. The Drug Enforcement Agency regulates the manufacture and sale of drugs and food products.

_____

_____

_____

_____

43. On a written prescription, the subscription section provides the name of the medication, the desired form, and strength of the drug.

_____

_____

_____

_____

44. Potentiation means that two drugs work together and synergism is an effect in which one drug makes the other less effective.

_____

_____

_____

_____

45. Diuretic medications dilate the bronchi in the lungs.

_____

_____

_____

_____

MULTIPLE CHOICE

Directions: Choose the best answer for each question.

46. The vastus lateralis injection site is located:

    a. on the upper arm.
    b. on the thigh.
    c. on the posterior buttocks area.
    d. on the lateral side of the hip.
    e. on the forearm.

47. The purpose of a DEA number is to:

    a. allow a physician to order all medications.
    b. provide insurance information for payment of prescriptions.
    c. track the prescriptions written for controlled substances.
    d. allow generic drugs to be substituted for brand name drugs.
    e. track the number of refills a patient can receive.

48. Which of these is a parenteral method of administering a medication?

    a. Injection
    b. Sublingual
    c. Instillation
    d. Buccal
    e. Inhalation

49. An undesirable side effect of a particular drug is:

    a. a teratogenic indication.
    b. a therapeutic response.
    c. an indication.
    d. a contraindication.
    e. an adverse reaction.

50. MAO inhibitor medications are indicated for the treatment of:

    a. high blood pressure.
    b. anemia.
    c. seizures.
    d. depression.
    e. high cholesterol.

51. Which of these drugs is prescribed to thin the blood?

    a. Tetracycline
    b. Lipitor
    c. Coumadin
    d. Codeine
    e. Valium

52. Which of these drugs is classified a Schedule I drug?

    a. Codeine
    b. Amphetamine
    c. Morphine
    d. Valium
    e. Marijuana

53. If a patient is required to take a teaspoon of liquid medication, the prescription would have the abbreviation:

    a. tb
    b. tid
    c. tbsp
    d. tsp
    e. tbs

54. Which of these is a drug that is typically prepared from an animal protein?

    a. Milk of magnesia
    b. Insulin
    c. Morphine
    d. Codeine
    e. Digitalis

55. Which of these drug classifications includes medications that induce sleep?

    a. Sedatives
    b. Stimulants
    c. Emetics
    d. Diuretics
    e. Antilipemics

56. Aspirin and ibuprofen are classified as:

    a. antihypertensives.
    b. anti-inflammatory agents.
    c. antihistamines.
    d. antibiotics.
    e. adrenergic agents.

57. Which of these represents the appropriate medication amount, needle gauge, and length for a deltoid injection?

    a. 0.5 mL, 18 g, 5/8″
    b. 0.5 mL, 21 g, 5/8″
    c. 1 mL, 18 g, 5/8″
    d. 1 mL, 21 g, 1″
    e. 2 mL, 21 g, 1″

58. Which method of medication administration would have the fastest action in the body?

    a. Subcutaneous
    b. Buccal
    c. Sublingual
    d. Intramuscular
    e. Intravenous

59. After issued by a physician, what is the maximum time a prescription must be filled?

    a. 2 months
    b. 4 months
    c. 6 months
    d. 30 days
    e. 90 days

60. The purpose of the Controlled Substances Act is to:

    a. regulate the manufacture and distribution of dangerous drugs.
    b. require drug companies to test all drugs to prove their effectiveness.
    c. regulate the manufacture and sale of drugs and food products.
    d. require all trade name drugs to be registered by the U.S. Patent Office.
    e. require physicians to write a prescription for all drugs.

61. Xanax and valium are classified as:

    a. antianginal agents.
    b. antianxiety agents.
    c. antiarrhythmics.
    d. anticonvulsants.
    e. antiemetic agents.

62. Which of these represents the correct angle of injection of a TB test?

    a. 5 degrees
    b. 10 degrees
    c. 30 degrees
    d. 45 degrees
    e. 90 degrees

63. A TB test must be read within:

    a. 24 to 30 hours.
    b. 32 to 40 hours.
    c. 40 to 52 hours.
    d. 48 to 72 hours.
    e. 60 to 82 hours.

64. A physician orders an injection of Lasix 40 mg. The available medication is Lasix 80 mg/2 mL. How much is the patient given?

    a. 2 mL
    b. 1.5 mL
    c. 1 mL
    d. 0.5 mL
    e. 0.25 mL

65. Which of these describes an emulsion?

    a. It is a tablet form of medication that dissolves high in the GI tract.
    b. It is a medication that dissolves over time rather than all at once.
    c. It is a medication inside a gelatin capsule.
    d. The medication is dissolved in alcohol and flavored.
    e. It is a medication combined with water and oil.

BRIEF EXPLANATIONS

66. Explain the difference between a tablet and an enteric-coated tablet.

    _____

    _____

    _____

    _____

67. Describe the use of each of these classifications of medications.

    Analgesics: _____

    Hypoglycemics: _____

    Emetics: _____

    Diuretics: _____

68. Explain why there are various methods of administration of medications.

    _____

    _____

    _____

    _____

69. Why is it important for a patient to disclose all over-the-counter drugs they take?

    _____

    _____

    _____

    _____

70. Explain the process that offices use to track their inventory and use of controlled substances.

    _____

    _____

    _____

    _____

WHAT DO YOU DO?

71. Read the following scenario and respond to the questions with a short answer.

Celeste Werner's 5-year-old daughter saw the physician for a sore throat and fever. After obtaining a positive strep test, the physician ordered amoxicillin, an antibiotic, for the patient. Directions on the prescription required four (4) daily doses for 10 days. Two weeks later, Ms. Werner called to schedule a follow-up appointment for her daughter because she was still sick with fever and sore throat. Upon questioning the mother, the medical assistant discovered that the mother did not give all the medication as directed to the patient but instead shared the amoxicillin with the other children hoping they would not get sick too.

a. How would you respond to the patient when she discloses this information?

_____

_____

_____

_____

b. Why is it dangerous to give a person a prescription medication that is not intended for them?

_____

_____

_____

_____

c. How will you reflect or document the mother's comments in the patient's medical record?

_____

_____

_____

_____

PATIENT EDUCATION

72. Write a short narrative script that you can use to provide patient education explaining the care of the injection site after administering a TB skin test. The education information needs to include the patient follow-up to evaluate the outcome of the test.

_____

_____

_____

_____

INTERNET RESEARCH

Visit the Centers for Disease Control and Prevention Web site at www.cdc.gov and research the adult immunization schedule. What immunizations should an adult receive? How will a medical office monitor their patients to ensure immunizations are up to date?

_____

_____

_____

_____

_____

_____

Procedure 19-1 | Administering Oral Medications

Name: _____ Date: _____ Time: _____ Grade: _____

Equipment: Correct oral medication, a disposable calibrated cup, a glass of water, and the patient's medical record

Performance Requirement: Student will perform this skill with _____% accuracy not to exceed _____ minutes. (Instructor will determine the point value for each step, % accuracy, and minutes required.)

Performance Checklist

Point Value	Performance Points Earned	Procedure Steps
		1. Wash your hands and gather the supplies.
		2. Check the medication label and compare it to the physician's order. If necessary, calculate the correct dose.
		3. For a multidose container, remove the cap from the container. Touch only the outside of the lid to avoid contaminating the inside.
		4. Single, or unit dose, medications come individually wrapped. Open the package by pushing the medication through the foil backing or by peeling back a tab on one corner.
		5. According to your calculations and the label, remove the correct dose of medication.
		6. Solid medications—pour the correct dose into the bottle cap and transfer the medication to a disposable cup.
		7. Liquid medication—open the bottle and put the lid on a flat surface with the open end of the lid face up to prevent contamination of the inside of the cap. Palm the label to prevent liquids from dripping onto the label. With the opposite hand, place your thumbnail at the correct calibration on the cup. Holding the cup at eye level, pour the proper amount of medication into the cup. Use your thumbnail as a guide.
		8. Greet and verify the patient's name to avoid errors. Explain the procedure. Ask the patient about any medication allergies that may not be noted on the chart.
		9. Give the patient a glass of water to wash down the medication, unless contraindicated (as in the case of lozenges or cough syrup). Hand the patient the disposable cup containing the medication.
		10. Remain with the patient to be sure all the medication is swallowed. Observe any unusual reactions and report them to the physician.

(Continued)

| Procedure 19-1 | Administering Oral Medications (*Continued*) |

Performance Checklist

Point Value	Performance Points Earned	Procedure Steps
		11. Thank the patient and give any additional instructions as necessary.
		12. Wash your hands and record the procedure in the patient's medical record.

CALCULATION

Total Points Possible: _____

Total Points Earned: _____

Points Earned/Points Possible = _____%

Student completion time (minutes): _____

PASS   FAIL   COMMENTS:

_____

Student's signature _____ Date _____

Instructor's signature _____ Date _____

Procedure 19-2 Preparing Injections

Name: _____ Date: _____ Time: _____ Grade: _____

Equipment: Medication for the injection in an ampule or vial, antiseptic wipes, a needle and syringe of appropriate size, a small gauze pad, a biohazard sharps container, and the patient's medical record.

Performance Requirement: Student will perform this skill with ____% accuracy not to exceed _____ minutes. (Instructor will determine the point value for each step, % accuracy, and minutes required.)

Performance Checklist

Point Value	Performance Points Earned	Procedure Steps
		1. Wash your hands and gather supplies.
		2. Review the medication order and compare it to the label on the medication container.
		3. Calculate the correct dose, if necessary.
		4. Open the needle and syringe package. Assemble if necessary.
		5. Withdraw the correct amount of medication.
		6. From an ampule: Tap the stem of the ampule lightly to remove medication from the neck. Wipe the neck of the ampule where the break will occur with an alcohol wipe. Wrap a piece of gauze around the neck and snap the stem off the ampule. Dispose of the ampule top. Insert a filtered needle into the ampule with the needle lumen below the level of medication. Withdraw the medication. Discard the ampule. Remove any air bubbles from the syringe.
		7. From a vial: Cleanse the stopper of the vial with an antiseptic wipe. Fill the syringe with a small amount of air equal to the amount of medication to be removed from the vial. Insert the needle into the vial and inject the air from the syringe into the vial above the level of the medication. Aspirate, or withdraw, the desired amount of medication into the syringe. Remove the air bubbles. Remove the needle from the vial.
		8. Place the needle guard on a hard, flat surface. Without contaminating the needle, insert the needle into the cap and scoop up the cap with one hand.
		9. Medication is now prepared for administration.

(Continued)

Procedure 19-2 | Preparing Injections (*Continued*)

CALCULATION

Total Points Possible: _____

Total Points Earned: _____

Points Earned/Points Possible = _____%

Student completion time (minutes): _____

PASS   FAIL   COMMENTS:

_____

Student's signature _____   Date _____

Instructor's signature _____   Date _____

Procedure 19-3	Administering an Intradermal Injection

Name: _____ Date: _____ Time: _____ Grade: _____

Equipment: Medication for the injection in an ampule or vial, antiseptic wipes, a needle and syringe of appropriate size (TB syringe), a small gauze pad, a biohazard sharps container, clean examination gloves, and the patient's medical record

Performance Requirement: Student will perform this skill with ____% accuracy not to exceed _____ minutes. (Instructor will determine the point value for each step, % accuracy, and minutes required.)

Performance Checklist

Point Value	Performance Points Earned	Procedure Steps
		1. Wash your hands and gather supplies.
		2. Review the physician's order and select the correct medication. Check the order carefully against the medication label.
		3. Prepare the injection according to the steps in Procedure 19-2 Preparing Injections.
		4. Greet and identify the patient. Explain the procedure and ask the patient about any known medication allergies.
		5. Select the appropriate site for the injection.
		6. Prepare the site by cleansing with an antiseptic wipe. Use a circular motion, starting at the injection site and working toward the outside.
		7. Put on gloves. Remove the needle guard.
		8. Using your nondominant hand, pull the patient's skin taut. Stretching the patient's skin allows the needle to enter with little resistance and secures the patient against movement.
		9. With the bevel of the needle facing upward, insert the needle at a 10- to 15-degree angle into the upper layer of the skin.
		10. Inject the medication slowly; a wheal will form.
		11. Remove the needle and dispose the needle and syringe in a biohazard sharps container.
		12. Remove your gloves and wash your hands.
		13. Document the procedure, site, and instructions to the patient.
		14. Tell the patient when to return (date and time) to the office to have the results read.

(Continued)

Procedure 19-3 | Administering an Intradermal Injection (*Continued*)

Performance Checklist

Point Value	Performance Points Earned	Procedure Steps
		15. When patient returns for evaluation, read the test results. Inspect and palpate the site for the presence and amount of induration.
		16. Document the test results.

CALCULATION

Total Points Possible: _____

Total Points Earned: _____

Points Earned/Points Possible = _____%

Student completion time (minutes): _____

PASS   FAIL   COMMENTS:

_____

Student's signature _____ Date _____

Instructor's signature _____ Date _____

Procedure 19-4	Administering a Subcutaneous Injection

Name: _____ Date: _____ Time: _____ Grade: _____

Equipment: Medication for the injection in an ampule or vial, antiseptic wipes, a needle and syringe of appropriate size, a small gauze pad, a biohazard sharps container, clean examination gloves, an adhesive bandage, and the patient's medical record

Performance Requirement: Student will perform this skill with ____% accuracy not to exceed _____ minutes. (Instructor will determine the point value for each step, % accuracy, and minutes required.)

Performance Checklist

Point Value	Performance Points Earned	Procedure Steps
		1. Wash your hands and gather supplies.
		2. Review the medication order, select the correct medication, and compare it to the label on the medication container.
		3. Prepare the injection according to the steps in Procedure 19-2 Preparing Injections.
		4. Greet and identify the patient. Explain the procedure and ask the patient about any known medication allergies.
		5. Select the appropriate site for the injection.
		6. Prepare the site by cleansing with an antiseptic wipe.
		7. Put on gloves.
		8. Remove the needle guard. Using your nondominant hand, hold the skin surrounding the injection site in a cushion fashion.
		9. With a firm motion, insert the needle into the tissue at a 45-degree angle to the skin and the bevel of the needle facing upward.
		10. Remove your nondominant hand from the skin. Holding the syringe steady, pull the syringe (aspirate) gently. If blood appears, discontinue injection. If blood does not appear, you may continue with the procedure.
		11. Inject the medication by slowly pressing down on the plunger.
		12. Place a gauze pad over the injection site and remove the needle at the angle of insertion. With one hand, gently massage the injection site with the gauze pad, and with the other hand, discard the needle and syringe into the sharps container after engaging the safety device.
		13. Apply an adhesive bandage, if needed.

(Continued)

Procedure 19-4 | Administering a Subcutaneous Injection (*Continued*)

Performance Checklist

Point Value	Performance Points Earned	Procedure Steps
		14. Remove your gloves and wash your hands.
		15. Document the procedure, site, and results, as well as any instructions to the patient.

CALCULATION

Total Points Possible: _____

Total Points Earned: _____

Points Earned/Points Possible = _____%

Student completion time (minutes): _____

PASS   FAIL   COMMENTS:

_____

Student's signature _____   Date _____

Instructor's signature _____   Date _____

Procedure 19-5 | Administering an Intramuscular Injection

Name: _____ Date: _____ Time: _____ Grade: _____

Equipment: Medication for the injection in an ampule or vial, antiseptic wipes, a needle and syringe of appropriate size, a small gauze pad, a biohazard sharps container, clean examination gloves, an adhesive bandage, and the patient's medical record

Performance Requirement: Student will perform this skill with _____% accuracy not to exceed _____ minutes. (Instructor will determine the point value for each step, % accuracy, and minutes required.)

Performance Checklist

Point Value	Performance Points Earned	Procedure Steps
		1. Wash your hands and gather supplies.
		2. Review the medication order and select the correct medication.
		3. Prepare the injection according to the steps in Procedure 19-2 Preparing Injections.
		4. Greet and identify the patient. Explain the procedure and ask about any known medication allergies.
		5. Select the appropriate site for the injection.
		6. Prepare the site by cleansing with an antiseptic wipe.
		7. Put on gloves.
		8. Remove the needle guard.
		9. Using your nondominant hand, hold the skin surrounding the injection site taut with the thumb and index or middle fingers, or grasp the muscle producing a deeper mass for the injection in a person who is very thin with little body fat.
		10. Hold the syringe like a dart. Use a quick, firm motion to insert the needle into the tissue at a 90-degree angle to the surface.
		11. Remove your nondominant hand from the skin. Holding the syringe steady, pull back the syringe (aspirate). If blood appears, discontinue injection. If blood does not appear, you may continue with the procedure.
		12. Inject the medication by slowly pressing down on the plunger.
		13. Place a gauze pad over the injection site. Remove the needle at the angle of insertion. With one hand, gently massage the injection site with the gauze pad.

(Continued)

Procedure 19-5 | Administering an Intramuscular Injection (*Continued*)

Performance Checklist

Point Value	Performance Points Earned	Procedure Steps
		14. Apply an adhesive bandage to the site, if needed.
		15. Remove your gloves and wash your hands.
		16. Observe the patient for any reactions.
		17. Document the procedure, site, and results, as well as any instructions to the patient.

CALCULATION

Total Points Possible: _____

Total Points Earned: _____

Points Earned/Points Possible = _____%

Student completion time (minutes): _____

PASS   FAIL   COMMENTS:

_____

Student's signature _____ Date _____

Instructor's signature _____ Date _____

Procedure 19-6 | Administering an Intramuscular Injection Using the Z-Track Method

Name: _____   Date: _____   Time: _____   Grade: _____

Equipment: Medication for the injection in an ampule or vial, antiseptic wipes, a needle and syringe of appropriate size, a small gauze pad, a biohazard sharps container, clean examination gloves, an adhesive bandage, and the patient's medical record

Performance Requirement: Student will perform this skill with _____% accuracy not to exceed _____ minutes. (Instructor will determine the point value for each step, % accuracy, and minutes required.)

Performance Checklist

Point Value	Performance Points Earned	Procedure Steps
		1. Wash your hands and gather supplies.
		2. Review the medication order and select the correct medication.
		3. Prepare the injection according to the steps in Procedure 19-2 Preparing Injections.
		4. Greet and identify the patient. Explain the procedure and ask about any known medication allergies.
		5. Select the appropriate site for the injection.
		6. Prepare the site by cleansing with an antiseptic wipe.
		7. Put on gloves.
		8. Remove the needle guard.
		9. Rather than pulling the skin taut or grasping the muscle tissue as in intramuscular injection, pull the top layer of skin to the side and hold it with the nondominant hand throughout the injection.
		10. Hold the syringe like a dart and use a quick, firm motion to insert the needle into the tissue at a 90-degree angle to the skin surface, and insert the needle completely to the hub.
		11. Holding the syringe steady, pull back the plunger (aspirate). If blood appears, discontinue injection. If blood does not appear, you may continue with the procedure.
		12. Count to 10 before withdrawing the needle.
		13. Place a gauze pad over the injection site. Remove the needle at the same angle at which it was inserted while releasing the skin. Do not massage the area.

(Continued)

Procedure 19-6 | Administering an Intramuscular Injection Using the Z-Track Method (*Continued*)

Performance Checklist

Point Value	Performance Points Earned	Procedure Steps
		14. Engage the safety device and discard the needle and syringe into the biohazard sharps container.
		15. Apply an adhesive bandage to the site, if needed. Remove your gloves and wash your hands.
		16. Observe the patient for any unusual reactions.
		17. Document the procedure, site, and results, as well as any instructions to the patient.

CALCULATION

Total Points Possible: _____

Total Points Earned: _____

Points Earned/Points Possible = _____%

Student completion time (minutes): _____

PASS   FAIL   COMMENTS:

_____

Student's signature _____   Date _____

Instructor's signature_____   Date _____

| Procedure 19-7 | Applying Transdermal Medications | |

Name: _____ Date: _____ Time: _____ Grade: _____

Equipment: Medication, clean examination gloves, and the patient's medical record

Performance Requirement: Student will perform this skill with ____% accuracy not to exceed _____ minutes. (Instructor will determine the point value for each step, % accuracy, and minutes required.)

Performance Checklist

Point Value	Performance Points Earned	Procedure Steps
		1. Wash your hands and gather supplies.
		2. Review the medication order and select the correct medication.
		3. Greet and identify the patient. Explain the procedure and ask about any known medication allergies.
		4. Select the appropriate site for the medication and perform any necessary skin preparation.
		5. Open the medication package by pulling the two sides apart. Do not touch the area of medication.
		6. Apply the medicated patch to the patient's skin following the manufacturer's directions.
		7. Wash your hands and document the procedure, including the site of the patch.

CALCULATION

Total Points Possible: _____

Total Points Earned: _____

Points Earned/Points Possible = _____ %

Student completion time (minutes): _____

PASS   FAIL   COMMENTS:

_____

Student's signature _____ Date _____

Instructor's signature _____ Date _____

Procedure 19-8 | Instilling Eye Medications

Name: _____ Date: _____ Time: _____ Grade: _____

Equipment: Medication, sterile gauze, tissues, and gloves

Performance Requirement: Student will perform this skill with _____% accuracy not to exceed _____ minutes. (Instructor will determine the point value for each step, % accuracy, and minutes required.)

Performance Checklist

Point Value	Performance Points Earned	Procedure Steps
		1. Wash your hands and gather your supplies.
		2. Greet the patient and verify the patient's name. Explain the procedure. Ask the patient about any allergies not recorded in the chart.
		3. Position the patient comfortably in a lying or sitting position with the head tilted slightly back. The level of the affected eye should be slightly lower than the unaffected eye.
		4. Put on gloves.
		5. Using sterile gauze, pull down the lower eyelid to expose the conjunctival sac.
		6. Ask the patient to look up.
		7. Check the medication label for a second time to be sure it is the right medication for ophthalmic use.
		8. When using an ointment, discard the first bead of ointment from the container onto a tissue without touching the tip of the container to the tissue.
		9. Moving from the inner canthus (inner corner) outward, place a thin line of ointment across the inside of the eyelid. Twist the tube slightly to release the ointment.
		10. If using drops, hold the dropper about half an inch from the conjunctival sac, not touching the patient. Release the proper number of drops into the sac. Discard any medication left in the dropper to prevent contamination of the rest of the container.
		11. Release the lower eyelid. Ask the patient to close the eye and gently roll it to disperse the medication.
		12. Wipe off any excess medication with the tissue. Instruct the patient to apply light pressure to the opening in the eyelid where tears drain, for several minutes.
		13. Clean the work area, remove gloves, and wash your hands.
		14. Document the procedure.

Procedure 19-8 | Instilling Eye Medications (*Continued*)

CALCULATION

Total Points Possible: _____

Total Points Earned: _____

Points Earned/Points Possible = _____ %

Student completion time (minutes): _____

PASS   FAIL   COMMENTS:

_____

Student's signature _____   Date _____

Instructor's signature _____   Date _____

Procedure 19-9 | Instilling Ear Medications

Name: _____ Date: _____ Time: _____ Grade: _____

Equipment: Otic medication and cotton balls

Performance Requirement: Student will perform this skill with ____% accuracy not to exceed _____ minutes. (Instructor will determine the point value for each step, % accuracy, and minutes required.)

Performance Checklist

Point Value	Performance Points Earned	Procedure Steps
		1. Wash your hands and gather supplies.
		2. Greet the patient and verify the patient's name. Explain the procedure.
		3. Ask the patient to sit with the affected ear tilted upward. Adults: Pull the auricle (outer ear) slightly up and back. Children: Pull the auricle slightly down and back.
		4. Insert the tip of the dropper without touching the patient's skin.
		5. Ask the patient to sit or lie with the affected ear up for about 5 minutes after the instillation.
		6. If the medication is to be retained in the ear canal, gently insert a moist cotton ball into the external auditory meatus.
		7. Clean the work area and wash your hands.
		8. Document the procedure in the patient's chart.

CALCULATION

Total Points Possible: _____

Total Points Earned: _____

Points Earned/Points Possible = _____%

Student completion time (minutes): _____

PASS   FAIL   COMMENTS:

_____

Student's signature _____ Date _____

Instructor's signature _____ Date _____

Procedure 19-10 | Instilling Nasal Medications

Name: _____ Date: _____ Time: _____ Grade: _____

Equipment: Medication, tissues, and disposable gloves

Performance Requirement: Student will perform this skill with ____% accuracy not to exceed _____ minutes.
(Instructor will determine the point value for each step, % accuracy, and minutes required.)

Performance Checklist

Point Value	Performance Points Earned	Procedure Steps
		1. Wash your hands and gather supplies.
		2. Greet the patient by name and explain the procedure. Answer any questions the patient may have.
		3. Position the patient in a comfortable, recumbent position. Extend the patient's head beyond the edge of the examination table or place a pillow under the shoulders.
		4. Put on gloves. Administer the medication.
		5. Instilling drops: Hold the dropper upright just above the nostril. Dispense one drop at a time without touching the patient. Keep the patient recumbent for 5 minutes to allow the medication to reach the upper nasal passages.
		6. Using spray: Place the tip of the bottle at the naris opening, without touching the patient's skin or nasal tissues. Ask the patient to take a deep breath; spray as the patient is inhaling.
		7. Wipe away any excess medication from the skin with tissues.
		8. Clean the work area, remove your gloves, and wash your hands.
		9. Record the procedure in the patient's chart.

CALCULATION

Total Points Possible: _____

Total Points Earned: _____

Points Earned/Points Possible = _____%

Student completion time (minutes): _____

PASS   FAIL   COMMENTS:

_____

Student's signature _____ Date _____

Instructor's signature _____ Date _____

20 Diagnostic Testing

Chapter Objectives

- Explain the difference between radiolucent and radiopaque, using examples.
- List ways to protect patients and yourself from radiation hazards.
- Describe how to prepare patients for routine x-ray examinations.
- Discuss how to teach patients about contrast examinations.
- List the general steps in a routine radiographic examination.
- Compare and contrast fluoroscopy, MRI, and CT scans.
- List three typical uses for sonography.
- Describe the medical assistant's role in radiographic procedures.
- Explain how to handle and store radiographic film.
- Contrast invasive and noninvasive techniques for cardiological diagnosis.
- Describe the placement of electrocardiogram electrodes.
- Perform electrocardiography.
- Identify the main wave forms used for interpretation on an electrocardiogram tracing.
- Discuss three types of electrocardiogram artifacts and how to prevent them.
- Describe how to apply a Holter monitor.
- Define tidal volume and forced expiration.
- Perform basic respiratory testing.
- Briefly describe bronchoscopy and arterial blood gas tests.
- Explain how to teach a patient to use a peak flowmeter.

CAAHEP & ABHES Competencies

CAAHEP

- Prepare a patient for procedures and/or treatments.
- Schedule patient admissions and/or procedures.
- Perform within scope of practice.
- Perform electrocardiography.
- Perform pulmonary function testing.

ABHES

● Identify diagnostic and treatment modalities as they relate to each body system.
● Comply with federal, state, and local health laws and regulations as they relate to health care settings.
● Schedule of inpatient and outpatient procedures.

TERMINOLOGY MATCHING

Directions: Match the terms in Column A with the definitions in Column B.

Column A

1. _____ Artifact
2. _____ Cardiologist
3. _____ Cassette
4. _____ Contrast medium
5. _____ Dosimeter
6. _____ Dyspnea
7. _____ Echocardiogram
8. _____ Fluoroscopy
9. _____ Murmur
10. _____ Radiograph
11. _____ Radiography
12. _____ Radiologists
13. _____ Radiology
14. _____ Radiolucent
15. _____ Radiopaque
16. _____ Rhythm strip
17. _____ Spirometer
18. _____ Teleradiology
19. _____ Ultrasound
20. _____ X-rays

Column B

a. A special x-ray film holder
b. Process of making x-ray films
c. A medical specialty that uses different imaging techniques to diagnose and treat diseases
d. An abnormal signal that does not represent the electrical activity of the heart during the cardiac cycle
e. A device used to measure the amount of air that is breathed in or out
f. Physicians who specialize in interpreting x-ray images
g. Invisible, high-energy waves that can penetrate dense objects
h. Shortness of breath
i. Shadow-like images of internal structures processed on a type of film similar to photography film
j. Physician who specializes in disorders of the heart
k. Abnormal sound made as blood moves through the heart valves
l. A long strip recording the heart activity for a certain lead or combination of leads
m. A substance that temporarily changes the absorption rate of a particular structure to highlight a specific organ
n. Uses high-frequency sound waves, instead of x-rays, to create images of the body
o. A small device clipped to the outside of clothing that records the amount of radiation a person is exposed to
p. Substances that allow x-rays to pass through them
q. The electronic transmission of radiological images, such as x-rays and CTs, from one location to another
r. Image of the heart created by the sound waves
s. Uses a continuous beam of x-rays to observe movement within the body
t. Substances that do not allow x-rays to pass through them

DEFINING ABBREVIATIONS

Directions: Provide the specific meaning of each of the following abbreviations. Watch your spelling.

21. ABG: _____

_____

22. ALARA: _____

_____

23. COPD: _____

_____

24. CT: _____

_____

25. ECG: _____

_____

26. GI: _____

_____

27. MI: _____

_____

28. MRI: _____

_____

29. NPO: _____

_____

30. PAC: _____

_____

31. PACS: _____

_____

32. PAT: _____

_____

33. PET: _____

_____

34. PTCA: _____

_____

35. PVC: _____

_____

36. SOB: _____

_____

37. SPECT: _____

_____

MAKING IT RIGHT

Each of the following statements is false. Rewrite the statement to make it a true statement.

38. Pulmonary tests are used in the diagnosis of disorders of the heart.

_____

_____

_____

_____

39. In the anteroposterior projection for x-ray, the patient is erect facing the film.

_____

_____

_____

_____

40. An upper GI study uses a continuous beam of x-rays to observe movement within the body in "real time" and is displayed on a monitor so the body part and its functioning can be seen in detail.

_____

_____

_____

_____

41. Using a stethoscope, the physician palpates the sounds made as blood flows through the heart and the heart valves open and close.

_____

_____

_____

_____

42. Chest radiography is a graph of electrical activity of the heart from various angles.

_____

_____

_____

_____

43. A Holter monitor test is an ultrasound of the heart using sound waves generated by a transducer.

_____

_____

_____

_____

44. Sinus bradycardia is an abnormally rapid heartbeat of 100 to 180 bpm resulting in decreased ventricular filling and low blood pressure.

_____

_____

_____

_____

MULTIPLE CHOICE

Directions: Choose the best answer for each question.

45. Which of these is an electrical impulse that starts in the heart before the next expected beat?

a. PAC
b. PAT
c. PET
d. PTCA
e. MI

46. In the ECG tracing, the T wave represents:

a. contraction of the atria.
b. contraction of the ventricles.
c. the resting period of the heart before the next cardiac cycle.
d. the time period between the end of the contraction of the ventricles and the beginning of the resting period.
e. the electrical activity of the atria as they pump out blood.

47. The V_4 ECG lead is placed:

a. at the fourth intercostal space at the right margin of the sternum.
b. at the fourth intercostal space at the left margin of the sternum.
c. at the horizontal level of V_5 at the midaxillary line.
d. midway between V_3 and V_5.
e. at the fifth intercostal space at the junction of the left midclavicular line.

48. Which of these terms means a decrease in blood supply to an area of the heart?

a. Arrhythmia
b. Infarction
c. Hypertrophy
d. Ischemia
e. Embolism

49. A wandering baseline in the ECG tracing would indicate:

a. patient tremors.
b. loose electrodes.
c. electrical interference.
d. muscle movement.
e. improper grounding.

50. While wearing a Holter monitor, the patient should not:

    a. sleep.
    b. eat heavy meals.
    c. shower.
    d. exercise.
    e. smoke cigarettes.

51. Which of these tests uses sound waves to provide an image of the patient's heart?

    a. Echocardiography
    b. Electrocardiography
    c. Holter monitoring
    d. Fluoroscopy
    e. Magnetic resonance imaging

52. What allergy could be dangerous for a patient scheduled for an x-ray requiring the use of a contrast medium?

    a. Penicillin
    b. Milk products
    c. Peanuts
    d. Iodine
    e. Eggs

53. Which of these procedures creates a series of cross-sectional x-ray views of an organ?

    a. Fluoroscopy
    b. Cholangiogram
    c. Computed tomography
    d. Sonography
    e. Endoscopy

54. Which of these procedures uses a combination of high-intensity magnetic fields, radio waves, and computer analysis?

    a. CT
    b. SPECT
    c. PET
    d. ALARA
    e. MRI

55. Which of these involves balloon angioplasty?

    a. PAC
    b. PTCA
    c. PAT
    d. CT
    e. MRI

56. Which of these is not one of the most recognized side effects of radiation therapy?

    a. Blindness
    b. Hair loss
    c. Weight loss
    d. Loss of appetite
    e. Digestive disturbances

57. Which of these tasks is not within the scope of practice for a medical assistant?

    a. Placing x-ray film in the automatic processor
    b. Preparing a patient for an x-ray
    c. Helping with the positioning of a patient for x-ray
    d. Interpreting x-ray films
    e. Managing the inventory of x-ray supplies

58. What is a specific guideline established by the American Cancer Society regarding screening mammograms?

    a. Women should have the first screening mammogram at age 20.
    b. Women who do not have any symptoms do not need any mammograms.
    c. Women over the age of 50 should have a routine screening every year.
    d. Women between ages 40 to 49 should have routine screening every 5 years.
    e. Women over the age of 60 do not need any screening.

59. Which of these exams is an invasive procedure?

    a. Echocardiography
    b. Stress testing
    c. Holter monitoring
    d. Electrocardiography
    e. Cardiac catheterization

60. When the ventricles contract before the next expected beat, the patient will have these in the electrocardiogram tracing?

    a. PAC
    b. PAT
    c. PVC
    d. PET
    e. PTCA

61. If not treated immediately, death will result from:

    a. premature ventricular contractions.
    b. ventricular fibrillation.
    c. premature atrial contractions.
    d. paroxysmal atrial tachycardia.
    e. sinus tachycardia.

62. On standard ECG paper, each small block is:

    a. 0.5 mm.
    b. 1 mm.
    c. 5 mm.
    d. 10 mm.
    e. 20 mm.

63. In the ECG, Lead I is:

    a. a bipolar lead.
    b. an augmented lead.
    c. chest lead.
    d. precordial lead.
    e. unipolar lead.

64. Which lead shows the electrical activity from the left arm and left leg directed to the right arm?

    a. Lead I
    b. Lead II
    c. aVF
    d. aVL
    e. aVR

65. Which part of the ECG cycle does the P wave represent?

    a. Resting period of the heart
    b. Contraction of the ventricles
    c. Electrical activity through the ventricle
    d. Contraction of the atria
    e. End of the contraction of the ventricles

BRIEF EXPLANATIONS

66. Explain these terms related to heart function.

    Hypertrophy: _____

    Ischemia: _____

    Infarction: _____

67. Why would a physician order a rhythm strip during ECG?

    _____
    _____
    _____
    _____

68. Provide one corrective measure for each of these ECG artifacts.

    Wandering baseline: _____

    Somatic tremor:_____

    AC interference:_____

69. Why is it important for a patient to disclose all over-the-counter drugs they take?

    _____
    _____
    _____
    _____

70. Explain why a physician would order Holter monitoring for a heart patient.

    _____
    _____
    _____
    _____

WHAT DO YOU DO?

71. Read the following scenario and respond to the questions with a short answer.

    Milton Berg, a 65-year-old patient, is scheduled to have Holter monitoring performed. He does not understand why he needs this test done since he has had multiple blood tests, 12-lead ECG, and a stress test. While being fitted for the monitoring device, he asks the medical assistant several questions.

    a. How would you respond to the patient when asked why he needs this test done?

    _____

    _____

    _____

    _____

    b. The patient states that he will just go home and sit on the couch for the next couple of days until the test is done. How will you respond to this comment?

    _____

    _____

    _____

    _____

PATIENT EDUCATION

72. Write a short narrative script that you can use to provide patient education explaining the preparation prior to having an upper GI x-ray exam.

    _____

    _____

    _____

    _____

INTERNET RESEARCH

Visit the National Institutes for Health Web site at www.nih.gov and research heart failure. What are the causes and how does the physician diagnose this condition? What does the treatment involve?

_____

_____

_____

_____

_____

_____

_____

Procedure 20-1 | Performing a 12-Lead Electrocardiogram

Name: _____ Date: _____ Time: _____ Grade: _____

Equipment: ECG machine with paper and electrodes and antiseptic wipes

Performance Requirement: Student will perform this skill with ____% accuracy not to exceed _____ minutes. (Instructor will determine the point value for each step, % accuracy, and minutes required.)

Performance Checklist

Point Value	Performance Points Earned	Procedure Steps
		1. Wash your hands and gather the supplies.
		2. Greet and identify the patient and explain the procedure. Suggest that the patient use the restroom if necessary.
		3. Turn on the machine. Make sure the patient cable is connected and working well.
		4. Enter the appropriate data into the machine, including the patient's name or identification number, age, gender, height, weight, blood pressure, and medications.
		5. Ask the patient to disrobe above the waist and provide a gown for privacy.
		6. Assist the patient into a comfortable supine position, providing pillows as needed for comfort. Drape the patient for privacy.
		7. Prepare the patient's skin by wiping away skin oil and lotions with antiseptic wipes.
		8. Apply the electrodes against the fleshy, muscular parts of the upper arms and lower legs. Connect the lead wires securely according to the color-coded notations on the connectors.
		9. Apply the electrodes to the chest locations V_1–V_6. Connect the lead wires securely according to the color-coded notations on the connectors.
		10. Check the sensitivity, or gain, and paper speed settings on the ECG machine before running the test.
		11. Press the automatic button on the ECG machine to start the test. The machine will move automatically from one lead to the next.
		12. When the tracing is printed, you should check for artifacts and a standardization mark.
		13. If the tracing quality is good, turn off the machine. Remove and discard the electrodes.

Procedure 20-1	Performing a 12-Lead Electrocardiogram (*Continued*)

Performance Checklist

Point Value	Performance Points Earned	Procedure Steps
		14. Slowly assist the patient into a sitting position.
		15. Record the procedure in the patient's medical record.
		16. Place the ECG tracing and the patient's medical record on the physician's desk, or give it directly to the physician, as instructed.

CALCULATION

Total Points Possible: _____

Total Points Earned: _____

Points Earned/Points Possible = _____%

Student completion time (minutes): _____

PASS   FAIL   COMMENTS:

_____

Student's signature _____ Date _____

Instructor's signature _____ Date _____

Procedure 20-2 | Applying a Holter Monitor

Name: _____ Date: _____ Time: _____ Grade: _____

Equipment: Holter monitor machine, patient incident diary, adhesive tape, and patient gown

Performance Requirement: Student will perform this skill with _____% accuracy not to exceed _____ minutes. (Instructor will determine the point value for each step, % accuracy, and minutes required.)

Performance Checklist

Point Value	Performance Points Earned	Procedure Steps
		1. Wash your hands and gather equipment and supplies.
		2. Greet and identify the patient.
		3. Explain the procedure, including how to use and care for the Holter monitor. Remind the patient of the need to carry out all normal activities for the duration of the test.
		4. Explain the purpose of the incident diary.
		5. Ask the patient to remove all clothing from the waist up and to put on the gown. Drape patient appropriately for privacy.
		6. With the patient seated, prepare the skin using antiseptic wipes for electrode attachment.
		7. Expose the adhesive backing of the electrodes. Follow the manufacturer's directions to attach each one firmly in the specified sites.
		8. Check the security of the attachments.
		9. Position electrode connectors down toward the patient's feet. Attach the lead wires and secure them with adhesive tape.
		10. To ensure the monitor is working properly, connect the cable and run a baseline ECG by hooking the Holter monitor to the ECG machine with the proper cable hookup.
		11. Assist the patient in dressing carefully, with the cable extending through the garment opening.
		12. Plug the cable into the recorder and mark the diary.
		13. Give instructions for a return appointment to evaluate the recording and the diary.
		14. Record the procedure in the patient's medical record.

Procedure 20-2 Applying a Holter Monitor (*Continued*)

CALCULATION

Total Points Possible: _____

Total Points Earned: _____

Points Earned/Points Possible = _____%

Student completion time (minutes): _____

PASS   FAIL   COMMENTS:

_____

Student's signature _____ Date _____

Instructor's signature _____ Date _____

Procedure 20-3 | Performing a Pulmonary Function Test

Name: _____ Date: _____ Time: _____ Grade: _____

Equipment: Pulmonary function machine or spirometer with calibration syringe, patient mouthpiece, and noseclip

Performance Requirement: Student will perform this skill with ____% accuracy not to exceed _____ minutes. (Instructor will determine the point value for each step, % accuracy, and minutes required.)

Performance Checklist

Point Value	Performance Points Earned	Procedure Steps
		1. Wash your hands and gather equipment and supplies.
		2. Greet and identify the patient and explain the procedure.
		3. Turn the pulmonary function test machine on. If necessary, calibrate the spirometer using the calibration syringe, according to the manufacturer's directions.
		4. With the machine on and calibrated, attach the appropriate cable, tubing, and mouthpiece according to the type of machine used.
		5. Using the keyboard on the machine, enter the patient's name or identification number, age, weight, height, sex, race, and smoking history.
		6. Ask the patient to remove any clothing that may restrict the chest from expanding.
		7. Ask the patient to stand, breathe in deeply, and blow into the mouthpiece as hard as possible. The machine will indicate when the patient should stop blowing.
		8. During the procedure, coach the patient as necessary to obtain each reading. Three repetitions usually are required to obtain the patient's best result.
		9. After printing the results, properly care for the equipment. Dispose of the mouthpiece in the biohazard container.
		10. Wash your hands and document the procedure. Place the printed results in the patient's medical record.

| Procedure 20-3 | Performing a Pulmonary Function Test (*Continued*) |

CALCULATION

Total Points Possible: _____

Total Points Earned: _____

Points Earned/Points Possible = _____%

Student completion time (minutes): _____

PASS   FAIL   COMMENTS:

_____

Student's signature _____   Date _____

Instructor's signature _____   Date _____

Patient Education

Chapter Objectives

- List the five main steps in a teaching plan.
- Describe four different teaching strategies.
- List five conditions necessary for learning.
- Summarize Maslow hierarchy of needs and explain how to use it.
- Identify three factors that can promote learning.
- Provide instruction for health maintenance and disease prevention.
- Discuss four obstacles that can interfere with patient learning.
- Identify some considerations for adapting teaching materials to meet the needs of specific patients.
- Instruct individuals according to their needs.
- Identify community resources.
- List the recommended annual screenings for maintaining good health.
- List and describe the main food groups in the food groups system.
- Explain how to modify a basic diet to treat a medical condition.
- Define range-of-motion exercises and explain why they're used.
- Explain what to teach patients about herbal supplements.
- Identify different stressors associated with illness or disease.
- Describe three relaxation techniques for managing stress.
- Explain the role of the medical assistant in educating patients about substance abuse.

CAAHEP & ABHES Competencies

CAAHEP

- Instruct and prepare a patient for a procedure or a treatment.
- Instruct a patient according to patient's special dietary needs.
- Use feedback techniques to obtain patient information including reflection, restatement, and clarification.
- Use medical terminology correctly and pronounced accurately to communicate information to providers and patients.

- Coach patients regarding office policies, health maintenance, disease prevention, and treatment plan.
- Coach patients appropriately considering cultural diversity, developmental life state, and communication barriers.
- Develop a current list of community resources related to patients' health care needs.
- Facilitate referrals to community resources in the role of a patient navigator.

ABHES

- Teach self-examination, disease management, and health promotion.
- Identify community resources and Complementary and Alternative Medicine practices (CAM).

TERMINOLOGY MATCHING

Directions: Match the terms in Column A with the definitions in Column B.

Column A	Column B
1. _____ Assessment	a. What a patient should achieve at the end of patient education
2. _____ Denial	b. Tasks to help reach patient education goals; objectives are performed at different points in the program.
3. _____ Implementation	c. The process of gathering information in order to determine the patient's problem
4. _____ Learning goal	d. The process of finding excuses for thoughts or feelings that would otherwise be hard to accept
5. _____ Learning objectives	e. The process the mind uses to block uncomfortable or distressing ideas from conscious awareness
6. _____ Noncompliance	f. When a person rejects a fact that's painful or difficult to accept
7. _____ Rationalization	g. The process used to perform patient education, the actual teaching
8. _____ Repression	h. The patient's inability or refusal to follow a prescribed order

DEFINING ABBREVIATIONS

Directions: Provide the specific meaning of each of the following abbreviations. Watch your spelling.

9. AA: _____

_____

10. AAP: _____

_____

11. ADHD: _____

_____

12. CDC: _____

_____

13. FDA: _____

_____

14. OCD: _____

_____

15. ROM: _____

_____

16. USDA: _____

_____

17. USP: _____

_____

MAKING IT RIGHT

Each of the following statements is false. Rewrite the statement to make it a true statement.

18. During patient education, the medical assistant must treat each patient differently and with prejudice.

_____

_____

_____

_____

19. The best source for assessing the patient's need for patient education is their family members.

_____

_____

_____

_____

20. Lecture is a good way to present basic information to the patient; however, the patient needs to be actively involved in the lecture.

_____

_____

_____

_____

21. A discussion is a one-way exchange of information. It works well when teaching patients about lifestyle changes.

_____

_____

_____

_____

22. When documenting education, the medical assistant signature implies that they did the teaching but, if another staff member helped with the education, do not include that information in the patient's chart.

_____

_____

_____

_____

23. According to Maslow hierarchy of needs, a person at the bottom of the pyramid has satisfied all the upper level needs.

_____

_____

_____

_____

24. Basic human needs are not necessary before people can focus on higher needs, such as taking personal responsibility for their health.

_____

_____

_____

_____

MULTIPLE CHOICE

Directions: Choose the best answer for each question.

25. Which of these statements about Maslow hierarchy of needs is accurate?

    a. Everyone starts at the bottom of the pyramid.
    b. Everyone moves from the top to the bottom of the pyramid.
    c. Some people never reach the top of the pyramid.
    d. Basic needs are not necessary in order for good patient education to take place.
    e. A patient must be at the top of the pyramid before patient education is scheduled.

26. Patients learn best when they feel:

    a. anxious.
    b. distracted.
    c. guilty.
    d. relaxed.
    e. noncompliant.

27. Which of these is not an example of a psychomotor skill?

    a. Doing crutch walking
    b. Instilling eye drops
    c. Performing dressing changes
    d. Finger puncture to monitor glucose
    e. Understanding kidney function

28. Which of these is the most effective method of teaching most patients about the dangers of smoking?

    a. Give the patient a brochure to read at home.
    b. Show the patient photos of a smoker's lung compared to a nonsmoker's lung.
    c. Refer the patient to the American Cancer Society.
    d. Provide statistical data on smoking.
    e. Discuss the cost of smoking.

29. Which of these organizations is a good resource when providing nutrition education for patients?

    a. USDA
    b. OSHA
    c. FDA
    d. DEA
    e. CDC

30. The specific branch of medicine that is concerned with promoting health and wellness is:

    a. rehabilitative medicine.
    b. chiropractic medicine.
    c. preventative medicine.
    d. orthopedic medicine.
    e. pediatric medicine.

31. Which of these is an important technique when providing patient education?

    a. Present materials in written paragraph format for the patient to read.
    b. Keep the information general and not personalized for each patient.
    c. Diagrams are not beneficial to use since not all persons are visual learners.
    d. Avoid using medical terminology and abbreviations.
    e. It is inappropriate to direct patients to visit Web sites for information.

32. Which of these best describes the evaluation process for patient education?

    a. It is a way to determine if the patient learned the information presented.
    b. It is a consolidated list of the major teaching topics.
    c. It includes the process used to do the training.
    d. It provides a summary of the training and documentation into the patient's medical record.
    e. It measures the patient's progress after the education.

33. Which type of education method may be difficult for a patient with physical impairments?

    a. Psychomotor skills
    b. Verbal discussion
    c. Video presentations
    d. Reading brochures
    e. Completing surveys

34. Which of these is not one of the needs of Maslow hierarchy of needs?

    a. Security
    b. Belonging
    c. Expectations
    d. Self-respect
    e. Self-actualization

35. Which of these conditions would negatively affect the patient's ability to receive patient education?

    a. An appropriate environment for training
    b. Using only one method to present training information
    c. Having a knowledgeable teacher or trainer
    d. Providing appropriate equipment for training
    e. Introducing valid information on the education topic

36. What information is not necessary to document in the patient's medical record regarding patient education provided?

    a. Date and time of training
    b. How the information was taught
    c. Evaluation of the teaching
    d. Insurance billing information for the patient education
    e. Any follow-up training necessary

37. Which of these represents behavior of a noncompliant patient?

    a. Patient does not follow a prescribed medication order.
    b. Patient returns for follow-up visit with the physician.
    c. Patient schedules an appointment with recommended specialist physician.
    d. Patient adheres to a diet plan and loses 5 pounds in 1 month.
    e. Patient asks for further information regarding the use of a new medical device.

38. Which of these represents an open-ended question?

    a. Do you have any questions?
    b. Do you think this training plan will work for you?
    c. Can you return next Tuesday to follow up on the training?
    d. Did you refill your medication?
    e. Can you please describe the training that you received today?

39. Two-way exchange of information in a discussion format works best when:

    a. showing a patient a training video.
    b. demonstrating how to use a medical device.
    c. teaching patients about lifestyle changes.
    d. showing anatomical charts and posters to the patient.
    e. providing booklets and pamphlets for the patient to read.

40. Which of these would best help the patient to remember training information?

    a. Role playing
    b. Lecture presentation
    c. Video presentation
    d. Printed materials to read
    e. Visiting a Web site

41. Which of these is an accurate statement regarding learning objectives?

    a. They are not required for patient education programs.
    b. The medical assistant does not develop these.
    c. They are not measurable.
    d. They must be specific to each patient.
    e. They are not included in the documentation of training.

42. What is the first step in the assessment process for developing patient education?

    a. Talk with the patient.
    b. Review your own attitudes.
    c. Select training materials.
    d. Review the patient's medical record.
    e. Ask the patient when they can start the education.

43. Which of these is not one of the basic steps in effective patient education?

    a. Assessment
    b. Planning
    c. Implementation
    d. Documentation
    e. Reviewing

44. Which of these is among the most common uses of hypnosis?

    a. Smoking cessation
    b. Controlling diabetes
    c. Managing asthma
    d. Self-injection of insulin
    e. Avoiding stroke

45. Which of these would help a patient manage their hypertension?

    a. Bland diet
    b. Diabetic diet
    c. Low-fat diet
    d. Low-sodium diet
    e. Liquid diet

46. Which of these statements is accurate regarding saturated fats in the diet?

    a. They are the best choices for healthy eating.
    b. They are found in products made from plant sources.
    c. They are solid at room temperature.
    d. They reduce the risk of heart disease.
    e. They are hydrogenated fats.

47. Which of these are not among the food group categories?

    a. Grains
    b. Milk
    c. Fruits
    d. Oils
    e. Sugars

48. Which of these is a closed-ended statement?

    a. Point to your area of pain.
    b. Tell me a little about yourself.
    c. Explain how you plan your daily meals.
    d. Describe how you feel when you take the medication.
    e. Describe your headache.

49. Which of these illnesses would impair the patient's mental health or cognitive abilities?

    a. Diabetes
    b. Alzheimer's disease
    c. Asthma
    d. Lung cancer
    e. Cardiac disease

BRIEF EXPLANATIONS

50. Explain the difference between open-ended and closed-ended statements or questions. Provide an example of each.

_____

_____

_____

_____

51. Explain how each of these may interfere with patient learning.

    a. Illness and pain: _____

    b. Patient's age: _____

    c. Patient's educational background: _____

    d. Physical impairments: _____

52. Describe the ideal teaching environment for patient education. Explain why each part of the environment is important.

_____

_____

_____

_____

53. Explain why it is important to understand Maslow hierarchy of needs when planning and implementing patient education.

_____

_____

_____

_____

54. Explain what it means when a patient is noncompliant. Provide an example of a noncompliant patient.

_____

_____

_____

_____

WHAT DO YOU DO?

55. Read the following scenario and respond to the questions with a short answer.

Celeste Young is a 47-year-old patient diagnosed with uncontrolled diabetes. In addition to her current oral antidiabetic medication, the physician orders daily injectable insulin, home glucose monitoring, and patient education on diet control. The patient appears quite upset and angry that she has to go through all these things to manage her glucose. When the medical assistant begins to talk with the patient about starting these activities, she asks the patient when she can come back to the office to do the necessary patient education and training. The patient says she will have to think about it and will call back when she has time.

a. If you were the MA, how would you respond to this comment from the patient?

_____

_____

_____

_____

b. How would you approach the training for this patient? What methods would you use?

_____

_____

_____

_____

PATIENT EDUCATION

56. Write a short narrative script that you can use to provide patient education about how to stop smoking.

_____

_____

_____

_____

INTERNET RESEARCH

Visit the Centers for Disease Control and Prevention Web site at www.cdc.gov and research patient education topics. Select one topic and report the resources and information available to set up patient education programs. Are there specific methods recommended for training?

_____

_____

_____

_____

_____

_____

_____

Procedure 21-1   Implementing Individualized Teaching

Name: _____ **Date:** _____ **Time:** _____ **Grade:** _____

Equipment: Patient's medical record and physician's orders

Performance Requirement: Student will perform this skill with _____% accuracy not to exceed _____ minutes. (Instructor will determine the point value for each step, % accuracy, and minutes required)

Performance Checklist

Point Value	Performance Points Earned	Procedure Steps
		1. Review the physician's orders and clarify any questions you have before you begin.
		2. Identify factors that may get in the way of the teaching or learning process.
		3. Consult resources for the specific topic you are teaching the patient.
		4. Create a set of instructions you can give to the patient.
		5. After you have prepared your materials, greet and identify the patient.
		6. Explain the procedure to the patient in a logical, step-by-step manner.
		7. Show the patient how to perform the procedure.
		8. Ask the patient to return/show the demonstration.
		9. Provide feedback and positive reinforcement to the patient.
		10. Ask questions to check whether the patient has understood the information.
		11. Provide the patient with the prepared instructions and any other materials.
		12. Document your teaching in the patient's medical record using a formal teaching plan.

| Procedure 21-1 | Implementing Individualized Teaching (*Continued*) |

CALCULATION

Total Points Possible: _____

Total Points Earned: _____

Points Earned/Points Possible = _____%

Student completion time (minutes): _____

PASS   FAIL   COMMENTS:

_____

Student's signature _____ Date _____

Instructor's signature _____ Date _____

Procedure 21-2 | Identifying and Using Community Resources

Name: _____ Date: _____ Time: _____ Grade: _____

Equipment: Computer with Internet to access resources and patient's medical record

Performance Requirement: Student will perform this skill with ____% accuracy not to exceed _____ minutes. (Instructor will determine the point value for each step, % accuracy, and minutes required)

Performance Checklist

Point Value	Performance Points Earned	Procedure Steps
		1. Determine what types of resources will be most useful for the patients in your medical office.
		2. Compile a contact list of resources you can use to find out about community services.
		3. Contact the resources to determine what services they offer.
		4. Create a list of services available. Include addresses, e-mail addresses, Web sites (if available), and phone numbers.
		5. Store this master list on your office computer.
		6. Use this master list to create a list of services specific to your patient's needs. Answer any questions your patient may have about the services available.
		7. Offer to make contact with the service for your patient.
		8. Document in the patient's chart the information provided.

CALCULATION

Total Points Possible: _____

Total Points Earned: _____

Points Earned/Points Possible = _____%

Student completion time (minutes): _____

PASS   FAIL   COMMENTS:

_____

Student's signature _____ Date _____

Instructor's signature _____ Date _____

22 Medical Office Emergencies and Emergency Preparedness

Chapter Objectives

- Identify duties that may be required of a medical assistant during an emergency.
- List the key elements for a medical office emergency action plan.
- List signs that may indicate an emergency.
- Describe the general steps to take after identifying an emergency.
- Discuss the steps involved in the primary assessment of a patient in an emergency.
- Compare the two methods for opening an airway and explain when each is used.
- Describe the steps involved in cardiopulmonary resuscitation (CPR).
- Describe the purpose and use of the automatic external defibrillator (AED).
- Describe the signs, symptoms, and treatment of shock.
- Explain how to control severe bleeding from a wound.
- Explain how to classify burn injuries and how to assess the extent of a burn using the rule of nines.
- Explain the difference between sprains, strains, fractures, and dislocations, and the emergency treatment for each condition.
- Identify the early symptoms of heart attack.
- Explain the signs of seizure and how to manage a seizure patient.
- Identify the signs and symptoms of an anaphylactic reaction.
- List the information needed before calling a poison control center.
- Contrast hyperthermia and hypothermia and list the dangers of each condition.
- Discuss the difference between a psychiatric emergency and an emotional crisis.
- Describe the steps in managing a patient who has fainted.
- Explain how to control a nosebleed.
- Identify unusual patterns of illness or patient behavior that could suggest bioterrorism.
- Explain the use of heat and cold in emergency treatments and identify adverse reactions to watch for.
- Describe the steps to follow for weather-related emergencies.
- Discuss the importance of preparedness in a catastrophic emergency.

CAAHEP & ABHES Competencies

CAAHEP

● Identify safety techniques used in responding to accidental exposure to blood, other body fluids, and chemicals.

● Discuss fire safety issues in the office or clinic.

● Describe fundamental principles for evacuation of a health care setting.

● Identify critical elements of an emergency plan for response to a natural disaster or other emergency.

ABHES

● Recognize and respond to medical office emergencies.

TERMINOLOGY MATCHING PART 1

Directions: Match the terms in Column A with the definitions in Column B.

Column A

1. _____ Abrasion

2. _____ Allergen

3. _____ Amputation
4. _____ Anaphylaxis
5. _____ Anaphylactic shock

6. _____ Avulsion
7. _____ Bioterrorism
8. _____ Cardiogenic shock
9. _____ Contusion
10. _____ Defibrillation

11. _____ Dehydration
12. _____ Diaphoresis
13. _____ Ecchymosis

14. _____ Edema

15. _____ Epistaxis
16. _____ Hematoma
17. _____ Hemorrhage
18. _____ Hemorrhagic shock
19. _____ Hyperthermia

20. _____ Hyperventilation

Column B

a. Terrorist attack involving the deliberate release of biological agents used to cause illness or death
b. Swelling, collection of fluid in an area due to injury or inflammation
c. Excessive bleeding caused by damage to a blood vessel
d. A scratch or scrape on the skin's surface
e. A collection of blood under the skin or in damaged tissue, a bruise
f. Profuse sweating
g. Nosebleed
h. A substance that causes a person to have an allergic reaction
i. Severe, potentially life-threatening, allergic reaction
j. The process of using electric shock to restore normal heart rhythm
k. Blood leaks into body tissues due to trauma or injury
l. Loss of all or part of an extremity
m. A type of shock, which is an extreme form of heart failure occurring when the heart's left ventricle is so impaired and blood is not adequately pumped to body tissues
n. A bruise, resulting from blood pooling under the skin following trauma
o. Abnormally rapid breathing; respirations that are too fast
p. Type of shock produced from excessive blood loss
q. An excessive loss of fluid from the body
r. A general condition of excessive body heat
s. A wound with a flap of skin torn loose; the flap may remain hanging or tear off altogether.
t. A type of shock due to a severe allergic reaction requiring immediate medical intervention

TERMINOLOGY MATCHING PART 2

Directions: Match the terms in Column A with the definitions in Column B.

Column A

21. _____ Hypothermia
22. _____ Hypovolemic shock
23. _____ Infarction
24. _____ Immobilized
25. _____ Ischemia

26. _____ Luxation

27. _____ Melena

28. _____ Neurogenic shock
29. _____ Pressure points

30. _____ Rescue breathing

31. _____ Rule of nines

32. _____ Seizures
33. _____ Septic shock
34. _____ Shock

35. _____ Sprain
36. _____ Strain
37. _____ Subluxation

38. _____ Syncope
39. _____ Vasodilation

Column B

a. Life-threatening condition in which the body system begins to shut down
b. Blood in the stool
c. To secure in a manner that prevents normal movement
d. An injury to a muscle and supporting tendons
e. Abnormal electrical activity in the brain that might be due to infection, trauma, or high fever; causes uncontrollable muscle contractions
f. Specific places where you can press an artery against a bone; arteries located close to the surface of the skin
g. The end of a bone is displaced from its normal position in a joint, also referred to as dislocation
h. Dilation of blood vessels increasing blood flow to an area
i. A bone pulled from its socket, but all structures in the joint, such as ligaments and tendons, keep their proper relationships, also known as a partial dislocation
j. Method used to calculate the percentage of total surface area affected by a burn
k. Lack of blood supply resulting in a decrease in oxygen supply to a body part
l. Fainting, temporary loss of consciousness
m. Shock caused by a general infection of the bloodstream
n. Type of shock caused by a dysfunction of the nervous system following an injury to the spinal cord
o. An abnormally low body temperature
p. Obstruction of blood flow to an area
q. Used in emergency situations when the patient has a pulse however is not breathing adequately
r. Type of shock occurring from excessive loss of fluids
s. An injury to a joint capsule and supporting ligaments

DEFINING ABBREVIATIONS

Directions: Provide the specific meaning of each of the following abbreviations. Watch your spelling.

40. AAPCC: _____

_____

41. AED: _____

_____

42. BSA: _____

_____

43. CAB: _____

_____

44. CPR: _____

_____

45. EMS: _____

_____

46. LOC: _____

_____

47. MI: _____

_____

48. PASS: _____

_____

49. RICE: _____

_____

50. SOB: _____

_____

MAKING IT RIGHT

Each of the following statements is false. Rewrite the statement to make it a true statement.

51. In cases of minor emergencies, treat the patient until help arrives to handle the situation and transport the patient to a hospital emergency room.

_____

_____

_____

_____

52. Replace items used during an emergency at the end of each month.

_____

_____

_____

_____

53. CPR is the process of using electric shock to restore normal heart rhythm.

_____

_____

_____

_____

54. Dehydration caused by diarrhea, vomiting, or heavy sweating also can lead to hemorrhagic shock.

_____

_____

_____

_____

55. A contusion is a wound with a flap of skin torn loose; the flap may remain hanging or tear off altogether.

_____

_____

_____

_____

56. Chemical burns are caused by contact with hot liquids, solids, superheated gases, or flame.

_____

_____

_____

_____

57. A sprain occurs when the end of a bone becomes displaced from its normal position in a joint.

_____

_____

_____

_____

MULTIPLE CHOICE

Directions: Choose the best answer for each question.

58. Which of these is not a typical symptom of a person who has a dislocation?

   a. Pain
   b. Hemorrhage
   c. Deformity
   d. Pressure
   e. Limited movement

59. A simple fracture:

   a. does not completely break the bone.
   b. is a dislocation of a joint.
   c. does not break through the skin.
   d. may become infected due to broken skin.
   e. is a partial or incomplete break.

60. The purpose for immobilizing an injury is to:

    a. eliminate pain.
    b. allow faster healing.
    c. avoid infection.
    d. ensure range of motion.
    e. prevent further injury.

61. Four-point crutch gait is recommended for patients who:

    a. can put some weight on each foot.
    b. have greater upper body strength.
    c. cannot use a cane.
    d. are permanently disabled.
    e. need a faster gait.

62. Which of these organizations does not offer CPR training?

    a. American Red Cross
    b. American Heart Association
    c. American Health and Safety Institute
    d. American Medical Association
    e. National Safety Council

63. Which of these items is not found in an emergency medical kit?

    a. Activated charcoal
    b. Disposable gloves
    c. Sharps container
    d. Scissors
    e. Triangular bandage

64. The primary assessment of the victim is usually completed in less than:

    a. 15 seconds.
    b. 30 seconds.
    c. 45 seconds.
    d. 60 seconds.
    e. 90 seconds.

65. The artery used to check for a pulse on a child is the:

    a. aorta.
    b. brachial.
    c. femoral.
    d. carotid.
    e. radial.

66. Secondary assessment of a victim includes:

    a. checking for responsiveness.
    b. obtaining vital signs.
    c. evaluating airway.
    d. determining circulation.
    e. checking for respirations.

67. Respirations that are too fast are referred to as:

    a. hyperventilation.
    b. tachycardia.
    c. hypoxia.
    d. hyperthermia.
    e. apnea.

68. Which of these conditions would exist if a victim has pink skin?

    a. Inadequate oxygenation
    b. Increased bilirubin due to liver disease
    c. Airway obstruction
    d. Decreased blood flow to a body part
    e. Vasodilation due to increased blood flow

69. What is the immediate first aid for a victim suspected of having a cervical spine injury?

    a. Ask the victim if they are able to move their head without pain.
    b. Elevate the victim's head making it easier for them to breathe.
    c. Immobilize the head so the victim is unable to move their head.
    d. Turn the head from side to side to check for bruising or reason for the injury.
    e. Lift the victim's head to check for bleeding from the scalp.

70. Which of these is not a typical sign or symptom of shock?

    a. Low blood pressure
    b. Cool, clammy skin
    c. Pale, cyanotic skin
    d. Diarrhea with abdominal pain
    e. Rapid, weak pulse

71. Which type of shock is due to excessive dehydration?

    a. Neurogenic
    b. Hypovolemic
    c. Cardiogenic
    d. Septic
    e. Anaphylactic

72. Which of these is a wound with a flap of skin torn loose?

    a. Avulsion
    b. Abrasion
    c. Laceration
    d. Puncture
    e. Hematoma

BRIEF EXPLANATIONS

73. Explain the difference between a simple and compound fracture.

_____

_____

_____

_____

74. Provide an example of the cause for each of these types of burns.

    a. Thermal: _____

    b. Chemical: _____

    c. Electrical: _____

75. Describe the appearance of a first-, second-, and third-degree burn.

    _____

    _____

    _____

    _____

76. Explain why it is necessary to teach the patient the crutch gait best suited for their condition or injury.

    _____

    _____

    _____

    _____

WHAT DO YOU DO?

77. Read the following scenario and respond to the questions with a short answer.

    Michael Evans is at his medical office to receive his biweekly allergy shot. He has multiple allergies to grasses and trees. He arrives at the office during the lunch break when the physician is not in the office. The medical assistant explains to Michael that she cannot give him the injection unless the physician is actually in the office. The patient becomes angry because he took off work and spent his lunch hour to come to the office for the injection. He states that he has been receiving these allergy shots for months and has never had a problem.

    a. How would you help this patient understand why injections are not administered when the physician is not in the office?

    _____

    _____

    _____

    _____

    b. What documentation would you enter in the patient's medical record about this encounter?

    _____

    _____

    _____

    _____

PATIENT EDUCATION

78. Write a short narrative script that you can use to provide patient education about the purpose and application of RICE therapy to treat injuries.

_____

_____

_____

_____

INTERNET RESEARCH

Visit the Centers for Disease Control and Prevention Web site at www.cdc.gov and research seizure disorders. What information is available regarding generalized and focal seizures? What symptoms characterize each type of seizure?

_____

_____

_____

_____

_____

_____

_____

Procedure 22-1   Performing Eye Irrigation

Name: _____ Date: _____ Time: _____ Grade: _____

Equipment: Disposable, unpowdered gloves; sterile ophthalmic solution, drape, gauze, emesis basin, and tissues

Performance Requirement: Student will perform this skill with ____% accuracy not to exceed _____ minutes. (Instructor will determine the point value for each step, % accuracy, and minutes required.)

Performance Checklist

Point Value	Performance Points Earned	Procedure Steps
		1. Wash your hands and put on gloves (unpowdered) for infection control.
		2. Check the label for the solution three times; make sure the solution label states it is for ophthalmic use.
		3. Have the patient lie down with the affected eye down or sit with the head tilted so the affected eye is lower than the other eye.
		4. Drape the patient to protect the patient's clothing.
		5. Place an emesis basin against the upper cheek near the eye. You may ask the patient to hold it.
		6. Use clean gauze to wipe the eye from the inner canthus outward to remove any debris from the lashes that might wash into the eye.
		7. Separate the patient's eyelids with the thumb and forefinger of your nondominant hand. Hold the syringe in your dominant hand. To steady the syringe, you may rest it lightly on the bridge of the patient's nose.
		8. Keep the tip of the syringe about 1 inch from the eye. Gently irrigate from the inner to the outer canthus. Use gentle pressure. Do not touch the eye.
		9. Use tissues to wipe away any excess solution from the patient's face.
		10. Assist the patient to a sitting position and remove the drape.
		11. Document the procedure in the patient's medical record.

| Procedure 22-1 | Performing Eye Irrigation (*Continued*) |

CALCULATION

Total Points Possible: _____

Total Points Earned: _____

Points Earned/Points Possible = _____ %

Student completion time (minutes): _____

PASS   FAIL   COMMENTS:

_____

Student's signature _____   Date _____

Instructor's signature _____   Date _____

Procedure 22-2 | Performing Ear Irrigation

Name: _____ Date: _____ Time: _____ Grade: _____

Equipment: Otoscope, drape, emesis basin, irrigating syringe, warm water or otic solution, and gauze

Performance Requirement: Student will perform this skill with ____% accuracy not to exceed _____ minutes. (Instructor will determine the point value for each step, % accuracy, and minutes required.)

Performance Checklist

Point Value	Performance Points Earned	Procedure Steps
		1. Examine the ear by straightening the auditory canal (follow procedure for adult or child).
		2. View the ear with an otoscope to locate the foreign matter or cerumen.
		3. Drape the patient with a waterproof barrier or towel.
		4. Place an emesis basin under the patient's ear.
		5. Fill the irrigating syringe; make sure the solution is warmed to body temperature to prevent further discomfort or issues for the patient.
		6. With your nondominant hand, straighten the ear canal. With your dominant hand, place the tip of the syringe in the ear opening. Direct the flow of the solution up toward the roof of the canal.
		7. Continue irrigating for the prescribed period or until the debris or cerumen is removed.
		8. Dry the patient's external ear with gauze.
		9. Have the patient sit for a while with the affected ear down allowing the solution to drain.
		10. Inspect the ear with the otoscope to see if the debris or cerumen has been removed. If the patient is experiencing any pain during this procedure, stop and inform the physician.
		11. Document the procedure in the patient's medical record.

Procedure 22-2 | Performing Ear Irrigation (*Continued*)

CALCULATION

Total Points Possible: _____

Total Points Earned: _____

Points Earned/Points Possible = _____%

Student completion time (minutes): _____

PASS   FAIL   COMMENTS:

_____

Student's signature _____   Date _____

Instructor's signature _____   Date _____

Section V

Clinical Laboratory

23 Medical Assistant Role in the Clinical Laboratory

Chapter Objectives

- List the reasons for laboratory tests.
- Describe the medical assistant's role in the lab.
- Identify the kinds of labs where medical assistants work and describe what these labs do.
- List the various positions in a lab and the duties of each.
- Name each type of lab department and explain what it does.
- List the common equipment used in most small labs and the purpose of each.
- Identify the types of hazards encountered in a lab and summarize how to manage them.
- Recognize safety signs, symbols, and labels.
- Explain how OSHA makes labs safer.
- List the safe behaviors employees should practice in the lab.
- Identify the information included on safety data sheets (SDS) and the purpose of these sheets in a health care setting.
- Identify CLIA and explain how it affects lab operations.
- Describe how quality control affects lab operations.

CAAHEP & ABHES Competencies

CAAHEP

- Identify safety signs, symbols, and labels.
- Identify safety techniques that can be used in responding to accidental exposure to blood, other body fluids, needle sticks, and chemicals.
- Describe the purpose of safety data sheets (SDS) in a health care setting.
- Discuss protocols for disposal of biological chemical materials.
- Identify principles of body mechanics and ergonomics.
- Demonstrate proper use of eyewash equipment and sharps disposal containers.

ABHES

- Comply with federal, state, and local health laws and regulations as they relate to health care settings.
- Practice quality control.
- Dispose of biohazardous materials.

TERMINOLOGY MATCHING

Directions: Match the terms in Column A with the definitions in Column B.

Column A

1. _____ Aerosol
2. _____ Anticoagulant
3. _____ Blood-borne pathogens
4. _____ Caustic
5. _____ Centrifuge
6. _____ Cytology
7. _____ Graduated
8. _____ Histology
9. _____ Microorganisms
10. _____ Normal values
11. _____ Phlebotomists
12. _____ Plasma
13. _____ Quality assurance
14. _____ Quality control
15. _____ Reagents
16. _____ Safety data sheets
17. _____ Serum

Column B

a. Acceptable ranges for laboratory test results
b. A process that ensures the laboratory performance measures up to required standards
c. A machine that separates liquids into their different parts, uses centrifugal force, or spinning that exerts force outward
d. The liquid part of the blood with the clotting agents removed
e. Particles suspended in gas or air
f. Living organisms that are only visible with a microscope
g. A program of written policies and procedures to ensure labs are meeting CLIA standards
h. Describes a container used for measuring liquids that is marked with divisions
i. Corrosive or abrasive
j. Provides the manufacturer's instructions for how to store, handle, and dispose the chemical or substance
k. Prevent blood clotting in conditions caused by clot formation and blocked blood vessels
l. The study of tissues
m. Dangerous organisms that can exist in the blood, body fluids, and secretions of an infected person
n. Substance used to produce a test reaction
o. Obtain blood specimens from patients
p. The study of cells
q. The liquid part of the blood with the clotting agents

DEFINING ABBREVIATIONS

Directions: Provide the specific meaning of each of the following abbreviations. Watch your spelling.

18. CLIA: _____

_____

19. CMS: _____

_____

20. COC: _____

_____

21. FDA: _____

_____

22. NFPA: _____

_____

23. POC: _____

_____

24. POCT: _____

_____

25. POL: _____

_____

26. PPE: _____

_____

27. PPM: _____

_____

28. OSHA: _____

_____

29. QA: _____

_____

30. QC: _____

_____

31. SDS: _____

_____

MAKING IT RIGHT

Each of the following statements is false. Rewrite the statement to make it a true statement.

32. A physician office laboratory, also known as a referral laboratory, is a large facility resembling a factory.

_____

_____

_____

_____

33. The safety data sheet is necessary to accompany specimens to the off-site laboratory so that the lab will know the patient and physician information and the tests requested.

_____

_____

_____

_____

34. The microbiology department tests the blood for various types of cells and how many of each type are present.

_____

_____

_____

_____

35. Immunohematology is often a separate part of a chemistry department. The department testing involves measuring levels of both medical drugs and illegal drugs in a person's blood.

_____

_____

_____

_____

36. Virology and mycology are areas of testing within the serology department of the laboratory.

_____

_____

_____

_____

37. Plasma is the liquid part of the blood with the clotting agents removed. Blood is drawn into a red tube allowing the blood to clot before centrifuging the specimen.

_____

_____

_____

_____

38. A pipette is a shallow, covered dish filled with a substance that grows microbes in a specimen (culture).

_____

_____

_____

_____

MULTIPLE CHOICE

Directions: Choose the best answer for each question.

39. Which of these lab tests is a common preemployment test?

   a. Urine drug test
   b. Complete blood count
   c. Human immunodeficiency test
   d. Pregnancy test
   e. Sexually transmitted infection testing

40. Which of the following labs are required to do proficiency testing?

    a. Physician office lab
    b. Reference lab
    c. Labs who perform patient tests covered by Medicare
    d. Hospital labs that care for indigent patients
    e. Research labs for drug companies

41. Laboratory QC programs satisfy the standards required by:

    a. POCT.
    b. FDA.
    c. OSHA.
    d. CLIA.
    e. AMA.

42. Which of these terms is not required on a QC log in the laboratory?

    a. Date and time of control sample tests
    b. Expected results of control sample tests
    c. Results obtained from control sample tests
    d. Corrective action taken for testing of control samples
    e. Patient names for each test performed

43. In order to ensure labs comply with CLIA standards, which organization does unannounced visits to labs to inspect them?

    a. AMA
    b. CMS
    c. EPA
    d. DEA
    e. DES

44. Which of these represents a high-complexity laboratory test under CLIA standards?

    a. Erythrocyte sedimentation rate
    b. Urine pregnancy
    c. Fecal occult blood
    d. Manual cell counts
    e. Hematocrit

45. Which of these tests is within the scope of practice for a medical assistant to perform?

    a. Semen analysis
    b. Urine sedimentation evaluation
    c. Pinworm testing
    d. Wet mount for parasites
    e. Erythrocyte sedimentation rate

46. Which of these situations would not require processing an incident report?

    a. Accidental needle puncture with contaminated needle
    b. Patient medication error
    c. Patient fall in the hallway on slippery floor
    d. Patient says an injection hurt
    e. Visitor slips in the restroom and receives bruise on forehead

47. Which of these organizations requires the use of PPE?

    a. OSHA
    b. NFPA
    c. SDS
    d. CLIA
    e. FDA

48. When preparing patients for specimen collection, which of these is not necessary to include?

    a. The name of the test
    b. The type of specimen requested
    c. The cost of the laboratory test
    d. The purpose of the test
    e. How long it will take to receive results of the test

49. The reportable range is the:

    a. setting of calculation points from the instrument by processing solutions of known values.
    b. range of tests an analyzer, instrument, or procedure is capable of producing results.
    c. actual patient results of a laboratory test.
    d. normal values of a specific laboratory test.
    e. physician's expected results of a laboratory test.

50. A centrifuged microhematocrit is classified as:

    a. high complexity.
    b. moderate complexity.
    c. low complexity.
    d. minimum complexity.
    e. waived.

51. Which of the following would not be qualified to perform PPM?

    a. Physician
    b. Medical assistant
    c. Nurse practitioner
    d. Medical technologist
    e. Physician assistant

52. Which of these is characteristic of physician office laboratories?

    a. They do the same level of testing as reference laboratories.
    b. Highly qualified medical technologists are required to staff the laboratory.
    c. Medical assistants can interpret and analyze laboratory results in a POL.
    d. They primarily perform waived laboratory tests.
    e. The laboratory testing is cheaper than the same tests run in a hospital laboratory.

53. A safety data sheet tells the medical assistant:

    a. how to clean up a biological or chemical spill.
    b. how much the product costs.
    c. how to operate a fire extinguisher.
    d. how to reorder the product.
    e. how to vacate an office in the event of an emergency.

54. What equipment keeps microbiology specimens at a certain temperature usually close to body temperature?

    a. Refrigerator
    b. Microwave
    c. Incubator
    d. Autoclave
    e. Centrifuge

55. When operating a centrifuge, what is a critically important safety practice?

    a. Use a gloved hand to help stop the centrifuge.
    b. Maintenance is only required when a tube breaks in the machine.
    c. Centrifuges are not safe to use in physician office laboratories.
    d. Balance the centrifuge with equal tube sizes and level of liquid.
    e. Only urine should be spun down in a laboratory centrifuge.

56. Which of these is not required when caring for the microscope?

    a. Carrying with both hands
    b. Covering the microscope when not in use
    c. Using lens paper to clean ocular areas
    d. Washing your hands
    e. Wearing gloves

57. A person professionally trained to look for abnormal changes in cells, under a microscope is a:

    a. pathologist.
    b. cytologist.
    c. medical assistant.
    d. histologist.
    e. medical laboratory technologist.

58. One of the most common cytology tests is a:

    a. Papanicolaou test.
    b. cervical biopsy.
    c. breast biopsy.
    d. prostate smear.
    e. streptococcus A.

59. Which of these is not a common chemistry laboratory test?

    a. Glucose
    b. Cholesterol
    c. Hematocrit
    d. Blood urea nitrogen
    e. Electrolytes

BRIEF EXPLANATIONS

60. Explain the function of each of these laboratory departments.

    Bacteriology: _____

    Virology: _____

    Mycology: _____

    Parasitology: _____

61. List four (4) tasks that the medical assistant is responsible for in the physician office laboratory.

    _____

    _____

    _____

    _____

62. Explain the purpose of the safety data sheet. Describe how the medical assistant uses it.

    _____

    _____

    _____

    _____

63. Why does a medical assistant need to understand the care and use of a microscope?

    _____

    _____

    _____

    _____

64. What is the function of the toxicology department of a hospital? What type of testing is performed?

    _____

    _____

    _____

    _____

WHAT DO YOU DO?

65. Read the following scenario and respond to the questions with a short answer.

    The office manager would like the medical assistant to start performing high-complexity laboratory testing on the new chemistry analyzer. A certified medical technologist manages the lab and agrees to train the medical assistant in the performance of the tests.

    a. If you were the medical assistant, what is the problem with this request?

    _____

    _____

    _____

    _____

    b. How would you respond to the office manager and the medical technologist?

    _____

    _____

    _____

    _____

PATIENT EDUCATION

66. Write a short narrative script that you can use to provide patient education explaining the collection of a urine specimen for a preemployment drug test.

    _____

    _____

    _____

    _____

INTERNET RESEARCH

Visit the Department of Labor Web site at www.dol.gov and research chain of custody drug testing. What are some of their guidelines for alcohol and drug testing?

_____

_____

_____

_____

_____

_____

_____

Procedure 23-1   Maintaining the Chain of Custody for Urine Collection

Name: _____ Date: _____ Time: _____ Grade: _____

Equipment: Tamper-proof collection container and transport bag, chain of custody forms, and patient's picture ID.

Performance Requirement: Student will perform this skill with ____% accuracy not to exceed _____ minutes. (Instructor will determine the point value for each step, % accuracy, and minutes required.)

Performance Checklist

Point Value	Performance Points Earned	Procedure Steps
		1. Greet the patient and obtain a picture ID.
		2. Have the patient empty his pockets before collecting the specimen.
		3. Turn off the water supply in the restroom used for collection. Add dye to toilet water to prevent the patient from using it as the specimen.
		4. Ask the patient to wash their hands prior to the collection to ensure there is no soap residue that would affect the specimen quality.
		5. Record the collection of the specimen and the name of the witness, if there was one present during the collection.
		6. Record the specimen's temperature (90.5°F to 99.8°F is acceptable). The minimum volume collected should be 35 mL.
		7. Have the subject and the collector sign the COC form, with the date and time of collection.
		8. Sign and attach tamper seals to each side of the container, going across the lid.
		9. Put the specimen and COC form in a tamper-proof bag.
		10. Seal the bag for transport to the testing facility department.
		11. Document the procedure in the patient's medical record.

| Procedure 23-1 | Maintaining the Chain of Custody for Urine Collection (*Continued*) |

CALCULATION

Total Points Possible: _____

Total Points Earned: _____

Points Earned/Points Possible = _____ %

Student completion time (minutes): _____

PASS   FAIL   COMMENTS:

_____

Student's signature _____ Date _____

Instructor's signature _____ Date _____

Chapter Objectives

- List the components of blood.
- Explain the functions of the three types of blood cells.
- Describe the role of the hematology lab.
- Identify the leukocytes normally seen in the blood and explain their functions.
- List the different tests in a complete blood count.
- Specify the normal ranges for each test in a complete blood count.
- Understand process for preparing a peripheral blood smear.
- Describe the structure of red blood cells and explain the tests that are performed on the cells.
- Describe the various types of anemia and the cause of each.
- Understand the process for performing a manual microhematocrit determination.
- Perform a manual hemoglobin determination.
- Understand the process for determining erythrocyte sedimentation rate using the Westergren method.
- Explain the functions of platelets.
- Explain the process of how blood clots form in the body and describe the tests that measure the ability to form clots.

CAAHEP & ABHES Competencies

CAAHEP

- Identify CLIA-waived tests associated with common diseases.
- Instruct and prepare a patient for a procedure or a treatment.
- Perform a quality control measure.
- Obtain specimens and perform CLIA-waived hematology test.
- Define basic units of measurement in the metric system.
- Analyze health care results as reported in graphs and tables.
- Reassure a patient of the accuracy of the test results.
- Differentiate between normal and abnormal test results.

ABHES

● Practice quality control.
● Perform selected CLIA-waived tests that assist with diagnosis and treatment.
● Perform CLIA-waived hematology testing.

TERMINOLOGY MATCHING

Directions: Match the terms in Column A with the definitions in Column B.

Column A

1. _____ Anemia

2. _____ Anisocytosis
3. _____ Erythropoietin
4. _____ Hematocrit
5. _____ Hematology

6. _____ Hematopoiesis
7. _____ Hemoglobin
8. _____ Hemostasis
9. _____ Leukemia
10. _____ Leukocytosis
11. _____ Leukopenia
12. _____ Neutropenia

13. _____ Neutrophilia
14. _____ Poikilocytosis
15. _____ Thrombocytopenia

16. _____ Thrombocytosis

Column B

a. The part of the red blood cell that binds oxygen and carbon dioxide
b. A low number of neutrophils
c. Variations in the size of a blood cell
d. The process of blood cell production
e. Condition resulting from reduced numbers of RBCs in the blood or decreased hemoglobin
f. Too few platelets
g. Too many WBCs in the body
h. Percentage of RBCs in whole blood
i. An increase in the percentage of neutrophils
j. Too few WBCs in the body
k. To control bleeding or stop flow of blood from the body
l. Hormone that is released from the kidneys and influences the production of RBCs
m. Too many platelets
n. Condition of irregular shape of RBCs
o. Disease in which unusually high numbers of abnormal WBCs are produced
p. The study of blood, blood-forming tissues, and blood diseases

DEFINING ABBREVIATIONS

Directions: Provide the specific meaning of each of the following abbreviations. Watch your spelling.

17. CBC: _____

_____

18. CLIA: _____

_____

19. ESR: _____

_____

20. HCT: _____

_____

21. HBG: _____

_____

22. MCH: _____

_____

23. MCV: _____

_____

24. PT: _____

_____

25. PTT: _____

_____

26. PT/INR: _____

_____

27. RBC: _____

_____

28. WBC: _____

_____

MAKING IT RIGHT

Each of the following statements is false. Rewrite the statement to make it a true statement.

29. Erythrocytes are the body's main line of defense against bacteria and viruses.

_____

_____

_____

_____

30. Nongranulocytes include platelets and erythrocytes.

_____

_____

_____

_____

31. Anemia is a disease in which unusually high numbers of abnormal WBCs are produced.

_____

_____

_____

_____

32. Neoplastic disorders involve problems with how food is used for nourishment and body repair.

_____

_____

_____

_____

33. The normal platelet range is 4,500 to 11,000/mm³.

_____

_____

_____

_____

34. Hyperchromia is a condition caused by reduced hemoglobin in the RBC and is associated with anemia.

_____

_____

_____

_____

MULTIPLE CHOICE

Directions: Choose the best answer for each question.

35. Which of these is not one of the five types of white blood cell?

    a. Neutrophils
    b. Platelets
    c. Lymphocytes
    d. Monocytes
    e. Eosinophils

36. A younger version of a neutrophil that is not fully mature is:

    a. a thrombocyte.
    b. an eosinophil.
    c. a band.
    d. a segmented neutrophil.
    e. a basophil.

37. In a differential count, the normal percentage of lymphocytes is:

    a. 5% to 10%
    b. 15% to 35%
    c. 35% to 40%
    d. 20% to 40%
    e. 50% to 60%

38. The function of the RBC is to:

    a. engulf bacteria.
    b. fight viral infections.
    c. produce vitamins.
    d. rebuild cell tissues.
    e. transport gases throughout the body.

39. Which vitamin is necessary to properly mature red blood cells?

   a. C
   b. B_{12}
   c. D
   d. E
   e. K

40. What type of anemia is caused from blood loss?

   a. Hemolytic
   b. Iron deficiency
   c. Pernicious
   d. Vitamin deficiency
   e. Hypochromic

41. A variation in the size of red blood cells is reported as:

   a. poikilocytosis.
   b. anisocytosis.
   c. hyperchromatosis.
   d. hypochromatosis.
   e. erythrocytosis.

42. The test that measures the percentage of red blood cells in whole blood is:

   a. hemoglobin.
   b. sedimentation.
   c. hematocrit.
   d. indices.
   e. thromboplastin time.

43. Which medication immediately inhibits the formation of blood clots?

   a. Heparin
   b. Penicillin
   c. Vitamin K
   d. Lasix
   e. Codeine

44. The two parts of whole blood are:

   a. white cells and red cells.
   b. granulocytes and nongranulocytes.
   c. formed elements and thrombocytes.
   d. plasma and thrombocytes.
   e. plasma and formed elements.

45. Hematopoiesis is the process:

   a. of separating the plasma from the formed elements.
   b. the body uses to manufacture bone marrow.
   c. the body uses to replenish hemoglobin.
   d. of blood cell production.
   e. the liver needs to make protein.

46. What best describes leukemia?

    a. It is a blood infection caused by bacteria.
    b. It is the result of low hemoglobin.
    c. It is a disease with an unusually high number of abnormal white blood cells.
    d. It is caused from a low T-cell count.
    e. It is treated with large doses of vitamin B_{12}.

47. The average percent of neutrophils is:

    a. 15% to 25%.
    b. 20% to 40%.
    c. 30% to 50%.
    d. 50% to 70%.
    e. 90% to 95%.

48. Which cell increases during an allergy reaction?

    a. Lymphocytes
    b. Eosinophils
    c. Thrombocytes
    d. Monocytes
    e. Neutrophils

49. What is the most likely cause of hypoxia?

    a. Lack of hemoglobin
    b. Bacterial infection
    c. Viral infection
    d. Low white cell count
    e. Parasite infection

50. What is the average life span of a red blood cell?

    a. 10 days
    b. 30 days
    c. 60 days
    d. 90 days
    e. 120 days

51. What is the main purpose of the hematocrit test?

    a. Determine the cause of infection.
    b. Evaluate the level of vitamin B_{12}.
    c. Determine the oxygen level.
    d. Detect anemia.
    e. Differentiate viral and bacterial infections.

52. The RBC measurement that determines the average red blood cell size is:

    a. MCV.
    b. MCH.
    c. MCHC.
    d. MCC.
    e. MHV.

53. An ESR reading of a female patient experiencing a significant amount of inflammation would be:

    a. 5 mm/h.
    b. 10 mm/h.
    c. 15 mm/h.
    d. 20 mm/h.
    e. 40 mm/h.

54. Which blood test can be performed on a handheld device?

    a. White blood cell count
    b. Hematocrit
    c. Hemoglobin
    d. Sed rate
    e. Platelet count

55. Which of these describes thrombocytosis?

    a. It would be a platelet count of 75,000/mm^3.
    b. It is a condition of too many platelets.
    c. It is associated with increased bleeding time.
    d. It would result in a platelet count of 100,000 g/dL.
    e. It is a condition of too few thrombocytes.

56. Which of these is a test designed to measure clotting time?

    a. Hematocrit
    b. Hemoglobin
    c. Sedimentation rate
    d. Prothrombin time
    e. Coumadin level

57. What is the meaning of hemostasis?

    a. Control bleeding or stop flow of blood.
    b. Increase the number of platelets.
    c. Cause vasodilation.
    d. Increase flow of oxygen.
    e. Increase bleeding time.

58. The prefix milli means:

    a. one-tenth.
    b. one-hundredth
    c. one-thousandth
    d. one-billionth
    e. one million times

59. Which of these blood tests is not included in a complete blood count?

    a. White blood count
    b. Red blood count
    c. Hemoglobin
    d. Hematocrit
    e. Sedimentation rate

60. A patient with a low platelet count should avoid taking:

    a. Tylenol.
    b. penicillin.
    c. aspirin.
    d. vitamin B$_{12}$.
    e. vitamin C.

61. A variation in the size of red blood cells is:

    a. hypochromia.
    b. hyperchromia.
    c. polychromia.
    d. anisocytosis.
    e. poikilocytosis.

BRIEF EXPLANATIONS

62. Complete the following chart providing the information requested.

Blood Test	Normal Value or Range for Male and Female
White blood cell count	
Red blood cell count	
Hematocrit	
Hemoglobin	
Erythrocyte sedimentation rate	

63. Explain the purpose of an ESR. What condition might be present if the level is too high?

    _____

    _____

    _____

    _____

64. What is the primary function for each of the white blood cells?

    Neutrophils: _____

    Basophils: _____

    Eosinophils: _____

    Lymphocytes: _____

    Monocytes: _____

65. Explain the purpose for a differential white blood count.

    _____

    _____

    _____

    _____

66. Explain why it is important to measure the size and color of the red blood cells.

_____

_____

_____

_____

67. What are two types of anemia and the cause of each?

_____

_____

_____

_____

WHAT DO YOU DO?

68. Read the following scenario and respond to the questions with a short answer.

Cindy Spencer is a new patient of the medical office. The medical assistant is obtaining her chief complaint. The patient states that she seems to get sick all the time with sore throats and colds. After the physician examines her, he orders the medical assistant to draw blood to send to the lab for a CBC and ESR. While the MA is drawing her blood, she asks these questions. How would you respond to these questions?

a. The patient wonders why the physician ordered the tests if she only has colds and sore throat. How would you explain the need for these tests?

_____

_____

_____

_____

b. The patient wants to know why she does not have to be fasting for these blood tests. What would you tell her?

_____

_____

_____

_____

PATIENT EDUCATION

69. Write a short narrative script that you can use to provide patient education explaining the reasons why a good nutritional diet is good for healthy blood.

_____

_____

_____

_____

INTERNET RESEARCH

Visit the National Institutes of Health Web site at www.nih.gov and research sickle cell anemia. What is the cause of this condition? What are symptoms? What is the prognosis for a person with this condition?

_____

_____

_____

_____

_____

_____

_____

_____

Procedure 24-1	Making a Peripheral Blood Smear	

Name: _____ Date: _____ Time: _____ Grade: _____

Equipment: Disposable gloves, clean glass slides with frosted ends, a pencil, a well-mixed whole blood specimen, and a transfer pipette.

Performance Requirement: Student will perform this skill with ____% accuracy not to exceed _____ minutes. (Instructor will determine the point value for each step, % accuracy, and minutes required.)

Performance Checklist

Point Value	Performance Points Earned	Procedure Steps
		1. Wash hands, assemble supplies, and put on gloves.
		2. Use a lavender-top collection tube to obtain blood specimen from patient.
		3. Label the frosted end of the microscope slide with the patient's name or identification number.
		4. Place the slide on a flat surface or hold the slide flat between the thumb and first finger on your nondominant hand. Place a drop of blood 1 cm from the frosted end of the slide.
		5. Use your thumb and forefinger on your dominant hand to hold the second (spreader) slide against the surface of the first slide at a 30-degree angle.
		6. Move the spreader slide back until it is touching the drop of blood. Allow the blood to spread under the edge for a fraction of a second. Then push the spreader slide at a medium speed toward the other end of the slide.
		7. Allow the slide to air dry.
		8. Properly take care of or dispose of supplies.
		9. Remove your gloves and wash your hands.

CALCULATION

Total Points Possible: _____

Total Points Earned: _____

Points Earned/Points Possible = _____%

Student completion time (minutes): _____

PASS   FAIL   COMMENTS:

_____

Student's signature _____ Date _____

Instructor's signature _____ Date _____

Procedure 24-2 | Performing a Manual Microhematocrit Determination

Name: _____ Date: _____ Time: _____ Grade: _____

Equipment: Disposable gloves, blood specimen from capillary or venipuncture method, microcollection tubes, sealing clay, and microhematocrit centrifuge with a reading device or a separate microhematocrit reading card.

Performance Requirement: Student will perform this skill with ____% accuracy not to exceed _____ minutes. (Instructor will determine the point value for each step, % accuracy, and minutes required.)

Performance Checklist

Point Value	Performance Points Earned	Procedure Steps
		1. Wash hands and apply gloves.
		2. Use blood obtained from capillary or venous blood draw.
		3. From a capillary puncture, touch the tip of the capillary tube to the blood at the puncture site and allow the tube to fill to ¾ or the indicator mark on the tube.
		4. From a venipuncture, touch the tip of the capillary tube to the blood in the EDTA tube and allow the capillary tube to fill to ¾ or the indicator mark on the tube.
		5. Place your forefinger over the top of the capillary tube, wipe excess blood off its sides, and push its bottom into the sealing clay.
		6. Draw a second specimen in the same way.
		7. Place the tubes, with the clay-sealed end out, in the radial grooves of the microhematocrit centrifuge opposite each other.
		8. Put the lid on the grooved area and tighten by turning the knob clockwise. Close the lid. Spin the tubes for 5 minutes or as directed by the manufacturer of the machine.
		9. Remove the tubes from the centrifuge and read the results. Instructions on how to do this are printed on the device.
		10. Take the average of the two tube readings and report it as a percentage.
		11. Dispose of the microhematocrit tubes in a biohazard container.
		12. Remove your gloves and wash your hands.

Procedure 24-2	Performing a Manual Microhematocrit Determination (*Continued*)

CALCULATION

Total Points Possible: _____

Total Points Earned: _____

Points Earned/Points Possible = _____%

Student completion time (minutes): _____

PASS   FAIL   COMMENTS:

_____

Student's signature _____ Date _____

Instructor's signature _____ Date _____

Procedure 24-3	Performing a Westergren Erythrocyte Sedimentation Rate	

Name: _____ Date: _____ Time: _____ Grade: _____

Equipment: Whole blood sample collected in EDTA (<4 hours old), a Sediplast system vial prefilled with 0.2 mL of 3.8% sodium citrate, an autozero calibrated Sediplast pipette, a sed rate rack, and a disposable transfer pipette.

Performance Requirement: Student will perform this skill with ____% accuracy not to exceed _____ minutes. (Instructor will determine the point value for each step, % accuracy, and minutes required.)

Performance Checklist

Point Value	Performance Points Earned	Procedure Steps
		1. Wash your hands and assemble equipment and supplies.
		2. Put on gloves.
		3. Remove the stopper on the prefilled vial. Using a transfer pipette, fill the vial to the bottom of the indicated fill line with 0.8 mL of blood to make the required 4:1 dilution.
		4. Replace the pierceable stopper and gently invert several times.
		5. Place the vial in its rack on a level surface. Carefully insert the pipette through the pierceable stopper using a rotating downward pressure until the pipette comes in contact with the bottom of the vial. The pipette will autozero the blood and any excess will flow into the reservoir compartment.
		6. Invert the vial to get a good mixture of blood and diluent. Make sure the pipette makes firm contact with the bottom of the vial.
		7. Let the sample stand for exactly 1 hour and then read the numerical results of the erythrocyte sedimentation in millimeters.
		8. Read the result at exactly 60 minutes and record the results.
		9. Properly take care of or dispose of equipment and supplies. Remove your gloves and wash your hands.

Procedure 24-3 | Performing a Westergren Erythrocyte Sedimentation Rate (*Continued*)

CALCULATION

Total Points Possible: _____

Total Points Earned: _____

Points Earned/Points Possible = _____ %

Student completion time (minutes): _____

PASS   FAIL   COMMENTS:

_____

Student's signature _____   Date _____

Instructor's signature _____   Date _____

25 | Phlebotomy

Chapter Objectives

- Identify the main methods of phlebotomy.
- Identify equipment and supplies used in routine venipuncture and skin puncture.
- Understand the proper use of venipuncture and skin puncture equipment.
- List the major additives, their color codes, and the suggested order in which they are filled from a venipuncture.
- Perform venipuncture and describe proper site selection and needle positioning.
- Perform skin puncture.
- Identify complications of venipuncture and skin puncture and how to prevent them.
- Explain how to handle exposure to blood-borne pathogens.

CAAHEP & ABHES Competencies

CAAHEP

- Perform venipuncture.
- Perform capillary puncture.
- Practice standard precautions.
- Select appropriate barrier/personal protective equipment (PPE) for potentially infectious situations.
- Display sensitivity to patient rights and feelings in collecting specimens.
- Explain the rationale for performance of a procedure to the patient.
- Show awareness of patients' concerns regarding their perceptions related to the procedure being performed.

ABHES

- Collect, label, and process specimens.
- Perform venipuncture.
- Perform capillary puncture.

TERMINOLOGY MATCHING

Directions: Match the terms in Column A with the definitions in Column B.

Column A

1. _____ Antecubital space
2. _____ Anticoagulants

3. _____ Antiseptics
4. _____ Bevel

5. _____ Capillaries

6. _____ Gauge

7. _____ Hematoma
8. _____ Hemoconcentration

9. _____ Hemolysis
10. _____ Phlebotomy

11. _____ Skin puncture

12. _____ Syncope

13. _____ Tourniquet

14. _____ Vacuum

15. _____ Venipuncture

Column B

a. The slant end of the needle where the opening is located
b. A soft, flexible rubber strip wrapped around the arm to block the flow of blood in the veins; used during venipuncture to enlarge the veins
c. The rupture of the blood cells
d. The inside area of the elbow; location of veins preferred for use in blood collection
e. Use a hollow needle to puncture a vein to obtain a blood specimen
f. Blood leaks into body tissues due to trauma or injury; may occur during or after blood draw
g. Small blood vessels in the skin
h. Substance or medicine used to prevent blood clotting in conditions caused by clot formation and blocked blood vessels
i. Process of collecting blood from a vein
j. A space from which the air has been removed or evacuated. Evacuated tubes are used to collect blood during phlebotomy
k. Agent that blocks the growth of bacteria. Example is 70% isopropyl alcohol used to cleanse the skin
l. The size of an opening, or lumen. The larger the gauge number, the smaller the opening of the needle.
m. Pooling, increased collection of blood components, occurs from application of tourniquet for long time.
n. Piercing the skin with a sharp object for the purpose of obtaining a small blood sample
o. Fainting; temporary loss of consciousness

DEFINING ABBREVIATIONS

Directions: Provide the specific meaning of each of the following abbreviations. Watch your spelling.

16. CLSI: _____

_____

17. EDTA: _____

_____

18. HIV: _____

_____

19. mL: _____

_____

20. OSHA: _____

_____

21. PST: _____

_____

22. SST: _____

_____

MAKING IT RIGHT

Each of the following statements is false. Rewrite the statement to make it a true statement.

23. The FDA and CMS require wearing gloves when drawing blood.

_____

_____

_____

_____

24. The most common one used in blood collection to cleanse the skin is a 10% bleach solution.

_____

_____

_____

_____

25. The bevel of a needle refers to the size of its opening, or lumen.

_____

_____

_____

_____

26. Hemoconcentration is the rupture of blood cells due to using a small-gauge needle for blood draw.

_____

_____

_____

_____

27. Clot activators prevent the blood from coagulating or clotting in the Vacutainer tube.

_____

_____

_____

_____

28. When verifying the patient's identity prior to a venipuncture procedure, ask the patient to state their insurance company name and group number.

_____

_____

_____

_____

29. Label the evacuated tube prior to the blood draw with the patient's last name and date and time of draw.

_____

_____

_____

_____

MULTIPLE CHOICE

Directions: Choose the best answer for each question.

30. What evacuated tube color is used to obtain a blood specimen for a blood culture?

    a. Red
    b. Light blue
    c. Green
    d. Gray
    e. Yellow

31. Which agency recommends the order in which evacuated tubes should be collected?

    a. AMA
    b. CLSI
    c. CDC
    d. OSHA
    e. CLIA

32. When blood is not obtained in the evacuated tube and you think the bevel of the needle may be against the wall of the vein, what action should take place?

    a. Remove the needle from the vein.
    b. Pull back the needle.
    c. Back out the needle and reposition in another direction.
    d. Slightly rotate the needle half a turn.
    e. Decrease the angle of the blood draw apparatus pushing the needle upward.

33. Which of these sites is appropriate to perform a venipuncture?

    a. The arm with an IV inserted
    b. The tissue appears edematous.
    c. There is scarring from an old burn.
    d. There is bruise from prior blood draw.
    e. There is wrinkled skin from aging.

34. Which of these will cause hemoconcentration of a blood specimen?

    a. Patient opens and closes fist numerous times prior to the blood draw.
    b. Patient complains of pain with the blood draw.
    c. The site used is on the nondominant arm.
    d. A syringe draw is from veins on the back of the hand.
    e. Not allowing the venipuncture site to dry prior to the needle puncture

35. Which of these represents the proper application of a tourniquet?

    a. Do not leave the tourniquet in place for more than 2 minutes.
    b. Tie the tourniquet so the tails (ends) fall toward the draw site.
    c. Tie the tourniquet 3 to 4″ above the puncture site.
    d. A tourniquet is not required when the vein is visible.
    e. The tourniquet should be placed as close as possible to the site of the puncture.

36. Which of these is the first choice of veins for venipuncture in the antecubital area?

    a. Cephalic
    b. Median cubital
    c. Basilic
    d. Radial
    e. Ulnar

37. A heel-warming device is designed to provide a temperature that does not exceed:

    a. 98.6°F.
    b. 100°F.
    c. 102°F.
    d. 105°F.
    e. 108°F.

38. Which of these is test performed on infants using a filter paper filled with blood from a heel puncture?

    a. HIV
    b. Down syndrome
    c. Cystic fibrosis
    d. Polio
    e. Phenylketonuria

39. Why is it recommended to use a smaller size evacuated tube when drawing blood on a fragile vein?

    a. A smaller tube size will not likely cause the vein to collapse.
    b. Using a smaller tube decreases the amount of pain the patient will experience.
    c. Smaller tubes have a smaller gauge.
    d. Not as many tubes need to be drawn.
    e. Smaller tubes are easier to transport.

40. What is the largest evacuated tube size available?

    a. 5 mL
    b. 10 mL
    c. 15 mL
    d. 20 mL
    e. 30 mL

41. Why are tubes called evacuated tubes?

    a. The tubes have additives.
    b. The tubes are single use only.
    c. The tubes are unbreakable.
    d. The tubes are easy to change.
    e. The tubes have a vacuum.

42. A tortuous vein is one that is:

    a. blocked with a clot.
    b. twisted, not straight.
    c. easier to puncture for blood draw.
    d. found only in the legs.
    e. a vein of choice for venipuncture.

43. What is the largest needle gauge recommended for venipuncture?

    a. 20 gauge
    b. 21 gauge
    c. 23 gauge
    d. 25 gauge
    e. 27 gauge

44. Which of these evacuated tubes has no additive?

    a. Red
    b. Light blue
    c. Green
    d. Gray
    e. Lavender

45. Which of these causes typically hemolysis?

    a. Using a 21-gauge needle for blood draw
    b. Performing a venipuncture with a winged infusion set
    c. Using tubes with additives
    d. Vigorous shaking of specimens
    e. Centrifuging specimens to obtain serum

46. A hematoma results from:

    a. using a small-gauge needle to perform venipuncture.
    b. blood leaking into the surrounding tissues.
    c. removing the tourniquet too soon.
    d. drawing multiple tubes.
    e. accidentally hitting a nerve when drawing blood.

47. What is the primary purpose of prophylaxis following an accidental needle stick?

    a. To protect the office from a law suit
    b. To verify current status of immunizations
    c. To document the incident
    d. To comply with office protocol
    e. To provide protective treatment for the prevention of disease after possible exposure to pathogens

48. Which of these evacuated tubes contains EDTA?

    a. Light blue
    b. Yellow
    c. Lavender
    d. Green
    e. Red

49. The first thing to do if a patient feels faint during a venipuncture procedure is:

    a. try to calm the patient.
    b. remove the tourniquet and take out the needle.
    c. have the patient lower his head.
    d. put a cold compress on the patient's forehead.
    e. loosen the patient's clothing.

50. What is the first thing to do when there is a blood spill?

    a. Apply a disinfectant to the area.
    b. Complete an incident report.
    c. Notify the office manager.
    d. Secure the area to contain the spill.
    e. Locate a red biohazard bag for disposal of items.

51. The additive in a plasma separator tube is:

    a. heparin.
    b. sodium citrate.
    c. EDTA.
    d. silica.
    e. culture media.

52. Which of these is not a reason to perform a skin puncture?

    a. When only a few drops of blood is needed
    b. When collecting a small quantity of blood from an infant
    c. For patients with extensive burns and scarring
    d. To cause the patient less pain
    e. To perform point of care single drop testing

53. Which of these indicates a poor quality vein for venipuncture?

    a. The veins sufficiently engorged with blood.
    b. The vein feels like a rubber band beneath the skin.
    c. The vein is straight for 1 to 2 inches.
    d. There are no hematomas near the vein.
    e. The vein appears tortuous.

54. Why is it important to avoid drawing blood on the side of the body where a patient had a mastectomy?

    a. The patient will bruise easily on that side.
    b. There is usually an IV inserted in that arm.
    c. There is poor lymphatic circulation and an increase of lymphatic fluid.
    d. It is embarrassing for the patient.
    e. The tissue on that side is more sensitive.

55. What is the corrective measure when the needle may be too deep and has gone too far beyond the vein?

    a. Push the needle forward.
    b. Pull the needle back a little.
    c. Rotate the needle slightly.
    d. Change tubes.
    e. Discontinue the blood draw.

56. Which of these statements is true regarding the use of syringes for blood draw?

    a. Blood-filled syringes are easier to transport to the laboratory.
    b. Smaller needles can be attached to syringes than those used in winged infusion sets.
    c. Syringe method draws are less painful for the patient.
    d. Syringes cannot be used with winged infusion sets.
    e. Pull the plunger slowly and rest between pulls to allow the vein to refill with blood.

57. Why are large evacuated tubes not recommended for venipuncture from fragile veins?

    a. They will cause a hematoma.
    b. The patient will lose too much blood.
    c. It is more painful for the patient.
    d. It may allow a vein to collapse.
    e. Vein selection is limited.

58. What substance is used to clean a blood spill?

    a. 10% bleach solution
    b. Antiseptic
    c. Alcohol
    d. Soap and water
    e. Betadine

59. Which of these statements is correct regarding PST and SST blood tubes?

    a. The PST holds a larger quantity of blood.
    b. The SST is used with the winged infusion set and the PST is not.
    c. There is an additive in the PST and no additive in the SST.
    d. There is no difference between the PST and SST blood tubes.
    e. PST tubes collect serum and SST tubes collect plasma.

BRIEF EXPLANATIONS

60. List the equipment and supplies required for venipuncture using a multisample needle system. What is the purpose for each item?

    _____

    _____

    _____

    _____

61. Provide an example of each of these common errors and the corrective measure.

Misidentification of the patient: _____

Hemolyzed specimen: _____

Error labeling the specimen: _____

62. Describe how to palpate a vein to determine a good one to use for venipuncture.

_____

_____

_____

_____

63. What is the difference between plasma and serum?

_____

_____

_____

_____

64. What are two things that should be done differently for venipuncture on an elderly patient or an infant?

_____

_____

_____

_____

65. What are two considerations when selecting the appropriate blood tubes for a venipuncture procedure?

_____

_____

_____

_____

WHAT DO YOU DO?

66. Read the following scenario and respond to the questions with a short answer.

Selena Barnes is a new patient who needs to have blood drawn for a CBC and chemistry panel, which requires a lavender and SST tube. As the medical assistant is preparing to draw the patient's blood, the patient asks why it is necessary to draw so much blood.

a. How would you explain the need to draw two different tubes of blood?

_____

_____

_____

_____

b. This patient has not had a good experience with blood draw in the past. She says that every time, she ends up with a huge bruise where they draw blood. What can you say to reassure this patient?

_____

_____

_____

_____

PATIENT EDUCATION

67. Write a short narrative script that you can use to provide patient education explaining the venipuncture procedure. This would be used with a patient or young child who has not had blood drawn in the past.

_____

_____

_____

_____

INTERNET RESEARCH

Visit the Centers for Disease Control and Prevention Web site at www.cdc.gov and research information on needlestick safety and preventing blood-borne disease transmission during invasive procedures. What recommendations are provided to avoid needlesticks?

_____

_____

_____

_____

_____

_____

_____

Procedure 25-1	Obtaining a Blood Specimen by Venipuncture

Name: _____ Date: _____ Time: _____ Grade: _____

Equipment: Laboratory requisition form and tube labels, multisample needle, single-use tube holder or winged infusion set, evacuated tubes, tourniquet, sterile gauze pads, bandages, sharps container, 70% alcohol pad or other antiseptic, permanent marker or pen, and biohazard barriers such as gloves, impervious gown, and face shield.

Performance Requirement: Student will perform this skill with _____% accuracy not to exceed _____ minutes. (Instructor will determine the point value for each step, % accuracy, and minutes required.)

Performance Checklist

Point Value	Performance Points Earned	Procedure Steps
		1. Complete the requisition form indicating the lab tests ordered.
		2. Check the evacuated tubes to ensure that they are not expired.
		3. Greet and identify the patient.
		4. Explain the procedure and answer any questions.
		5. Put on disposable gloves.
		6. Assemble the multisample needle and tube holder.
		7. If using a winged infusion set, attach the apparatus to the tube holder or syringe. Extend the tubing of the winged infusion set to straighten it.
		8. Ask the patient to sit with a well-supported arm, straight or bent at a 15-degree angle at the elbow.
		9. Properly apply the tourniquet around the patient's arm three to four inches above the elbow.
		10. Ask the patient to make a fist and hold it. Do not allow the patient to pump the fist.
		11. Use your gloved index finger to palpate a vein. Then, trace the vein with your finger to determine the direction and depth of the vein.
		12. Release the tourniquet.
		13. Cleanse the venipuncture site with an alcohol pad using a circular motion starting from the center and working outward. Allow it to air-dry.
		14. Reapply the tourniquet using a half-bow knot.
		15. Hold the blood draw equipment with your dominant hand. Ask the patient to make a fist with their hand.

(Continued)

Procedure 25-1   Obtaining a Blood Specimen by Venipuncture (*Continued*)

Performance Checklist

Point Value	Performance Points Earned	Procedure Steps
		16. Grasp the patient's arm with the other hand and use your thumb to draw the skin taut over the site.
		17. With the bevel of the needle facing up, line up the needle with the vein about one-fourth to one-half inch below the site where the vein is to be entered. Insert the needle into the vein at a 15- to 30-degree angle. Remove your nondominant hand.
		18. Using a syringe, slowly pull back the plunger of the syringe allowing blood to flow into the syringe.
		19. Using an evacuated tube system, place fingers on the flange of the tube holder, and with the thumb, push the tube onto the needle inside the holder.
		20. When blood begins to flow into the tube or syringe, you can release the tourniquet and allow the patient to release the fist.
		21. Allow the syringe or tube to fill to capacity. When blood flow stops, remove the tube from the adapter.
		22. Place a sterile gauze pad over the puncture site as you are withdrawing the needle.
		23. Engage the safety device on the needle and immediately dispose of the needle and tube holder into the sharps container.
		24. Apply pressure or have the patient apply direct pressure for 5 minutes. Do not let the patient bend the arm at the elbow.
		25. If a syringe was used, transfer the blood from the syringe into the evacuated tubes using a blood transfer device.
		26. If the tubes contain an anticoagulant, you should mix immediately by gently inverting the tube 8 to 10 times.
		27. Check the puncture site and apply a dressing.
		28. Thank the patient and clean the work area discarding used and soiled supplies in appropriate containers.
		29. Remove your gloves and wash your hands.
		30. Process specimens to transport to the laboratory.
		31. Document the procedure in the patient's medical record.

Procedure 25-1	Obtaining a Blood Specimen by Venipuncture (*Continued*)

CALCULATION

Total Points Possible: _____

Total Points Earned: _____

Points Earned/Points Possible = _____%

Student completion time (minutes): _____

PASS   FAIL   COMMENTS:

_____

Student's signature _____   Date _____

Instructor's signature _____   Date _____

Procedure 25-2   Obtaining a Blood Specimen by Skin Puncture

Name: _____ Date: _____ Time: _____ Grade: _____

Equipment: Single-use skin puncture device, 70% alcohol or other antiseptic, sterile gauze pads, microcollection tubes and sealing clay or microcollection containers, heel-warming device (if necessary), and gloves, biohazard sharps container, and laboratory requisition form.

Performance Requirement: Student will perform this skill with ____% accuracy not to exceed _____ minutes. (Instructor will determine the point value for each step, % accuracy, and minutes required)

Performance Checklist

Point Value	Performance Points Earned	Procedure Steps
		1. Wash your hands and gather your supplies.
		2. Complete the laboratory requisition form.
		3. Greet and identify the patient, or if the patient is a child, confirm the identity with the parent or guardian. Explain the procedure and answer any questions.
		4. Put on gloves.
		5. Select the puncture site. Make sure the site chosen is warm. Gently massage the finger from the base to the tip to increase the blood flow.
		6. Grasp the finger or heel firmly with your nondominant hand. Cleanse the area with alcohol and allow to air-dry.
		7. Place the skin puncture device over the puncture site and activate the lancet.
		8. Wipe away the first drop of blood.
		9. Collect the specimen touching only the tip of the microcollection tube or container to the drop of blood.
		10. As each microcollection tube is filled, place it in sealing clay to cap the end of the tube.
		11. Once the blood collection is complete, apply pressure to the site with clean gauze or have the patient apply pressure.
		12. Perform the laboratory tests or prepare the specimens for transport to the laboratory.
		13. Thank the patient and clean the work area discarding used and soiled supplies in appropriate containers.
		14. Remove your gloves and wash your hands.
		15. Document the procedure in the patient's medical record.

| Procedure 25-2 | Obtaining a Blood Specimen by Skin Puncture (*Continued*) |

CALCULATION

Total Points Possible: _____

Total Points Earned: _____

Points Earned/Points Possible = _____%

Student completion time (minutes): _____

PASS   FAIL   COMMENTS:

_____

Student's signature _____   Date _____

Instructor's signature _____   Date _____

Chapter Objectives

- Describe the different types of immunity.
- Identify the different types of antibodies.
- List the reasons for immunological testing.
- Describe the antigen–antibody reaction.
- Explain the principles of agglutination testing and ELISA.
- Summarize the proper storage of handling of immunology test kits.
- Describe the ways that quality control is applied to immunology testing.
- List and describe immunology tests most commonly performed in the medical office or physician office lab.
- Perform an HCG pregnancy test.
- Perform a group A rapid strep test.
- Identify the major blood types and explain why differences in blood type exist.
- Describe how blood is typed and explain why this testing is important.

CAAHEP & ABHES Competencies

CAAHEP

- Perform patient screening using established protocols.
- Obtain specimens and perform CLIA-waived immunology test.
- Differentiate between normal and abnormal test results.
- Reassure a patient of the accuracy of the test results.

ABHES

- Practice quality control.
- Perform selected CLIA-waived immunology tests that assist with diagnosis and treatment.
- Perform selected CLIA-waived kit testing including pregnancy and quick strep testing that assist with diagnosis and treatment.
- Collect, label, and process specimens.
- Obtain throat specimens for microbiologic testing.

TERMINOLOGY MATCHING

Directions: Match the terms in Column A with the definitions in Column B.

Column A

1. _____ Active induced immunity
2. _____ Active natural immunity
3. _____ Agglutination
4. _____ Antibody
5. _____ Antigens
6. _____ Globulins
7. _____ Immunoglobulin
8. _____ Immunohematology
9. _____ Immunology
10. _____ Passive induced immunity
11. _____ Passive natural immunity
12. _____ RhoGAM

Column B

a. Group of proteins that make antibodies
b. A blood protein produced in response to and counteracting a specific antigen
c. Testing on red blood cells (RBCs) and serum or plasma to make sure that blood from a donor matches the blood of the person who receives it
d. Occurs when a person is exposed to a foreign antigen as part of therapy and develops his own antibodies to fight it
e. Occurs when a person receives already-made antibodies as part of therapy
f. Occurs when people are exposed to a foreign antigen as a natural process and develop their own antibodies to fight it
g. Protein-based antibodies of the immune system
h. The clumping together of materials that are suspended in a liquid
i. Rh immune globin injected when there is Rh incompatibility during pregnancy
j. Toxins or other foreign substances that induce an immune response in the body
k. Occurs when infants receive already-made antibodies from their mothers
l. A branch of medicine that focuses on the study of the immune system

DEFINING ABBREVIATIONS

Directions: Provide the specific meaning of each of the following abbreviations. Watch your spelling.

13. ELISA: _____

_____

14. HCG: _____

_____

15. HIV: _____

_____

16. RA: _____

_____

17. Rh: _____

_____

MAKING IT RIGHT

Each of the following statements is false. Rewrite the statement to make it a true statement.

18. Globulins are toxins or other foreign substances that induce an immune response in the body, especially the production of antibodies.

   _____

   _____

   _____

   _____

19. Receiving an MMR vaccination is an example of passive natural immunity.

   _____

   _____

   _____

   _____

20. IgG antibody actions are responsible for a severe allergic reaction called anaphylactic shock.

   _____

   _____

   _____

   _____

21. Enzyme-linked immunosorbent assays rely on clumping of cells to show positive or negative results.

   _____

   _____

   _____

   _____

22. When performing agglutination tests, a false negative is a result that says a substance is present in a specimen when it actually is not.

   _____

   _____

   _____

   _____

23. Mononucleosis is an autoimmune disease that affects the joints.

   _____

   _____

   _____

   _____

24. Pregnancy tests are based on detecting the luteinizing and follicle-stimulating hormones.

_____

_____

_____

_____

MULTIPLE CHOICE

Directions: Choose the best answer for each question.

25. Which organization maintains a list of current immunization schedules?

   a. FDA
   b. CDC
   c. EPA
   d. CLIA
   e. OSHA

26. Injecting RhoGAM into an Rh-negative mother is an example of:

   a. active natural immunity.
   b. active induced immunity.
   c. active acquired immunity.
   d. passive induced immunity..
   e. passive natural immunity.

27. Which of these is not a form of immunity?

   a. Active natural immunity
   b. Active induced immunity
   c. Passive natural immunity
   d. Passive induced immunity
   e. Processed induced immunity

28. The first immunoglobulin to appear when the body detects an antigen is:

   a. IgG.
   b. IgE.
   c. IgM.
   d. IgA.
   e. IgD.

29. Immunology is also known as:

   a. toxicology.
   b. blood banking.
   c. chemistry.
   d. microbiology.
   e. serology.

30. Immunohematology is the testing that blood banks do on:

   a. red blood cells.
   b. white blood cells.
   c. platelets.
   d. chemicals.
   e. hormones.

31. Which of these conditions is not determined through immunology testing?

    a. Mononucleosis
    b. Pregnancy
    c. Rheumatoid arthritis
    d. Syphilis
    e. Rubella

32. Which of these statements is true about storing reagents in test kits?

    a. Reagents must be refrigerated.
    b. Kits use reagents that remain at room temperature.
    c. Sunlight or direct light does not affect the quality of the reagents.
    d. Reagents may require room temperature or refrigeration.
    e. Reagent must be frozen to maintain effectiveness.

33. Which of these is not a good practice when using reagents?

    a. Reagents are effective at least 1 week beyond the expiration date listed on the kit.
    b. Write the date and your initials on a new test kit when opened.
    c. Read instructions for each new kit in case they have changed.
    d. Store reagents according to instructions provided by the manufacturer.
    e. Check expiration date on the kit box.

34. An autoimmune disease is one that:

    a. only affects patients with genetic problems.
    b. causes only10% of rheumatoid arthritis patients have a positive test for the rheumatoid factor.
    c. causes a person to produce antibodies against their own cells or tissue.
    d. does not affect elderly patients.
    e. comes on suddenly and then disappears.

35. Epstein-Barr virus causes:

    a. rheumatoid arthritis.
    b. strep infections.
    c. shingles.
    d. meningitis.
    e. mononucleosis.

36. Which of these hormones is detected in a pregnancy test if the woman is pregnant?

    a. Luteinizing hormone
    b. Human chorionic gonadotropin hormone
    c. Follicle-stimulating hormone
    d. Prolactin hormone
    e. Oxytocin hormone

37. The most common bacterial cause of a sore throat is:

    a. *Staphylococcus*.
    b. infectious mononucleosis.
    c. nasopharyngitis.
    d. group A *Streptococcus*.
    e. herpes simplex.

38. How long does it take to grow bacteria in a culture medium?

    a. 1 to 2 hours
    b. 4 to 8 hours
    c. 8 to 12 hours
    d. 18 to 24 hours
    e. 48 to 72 hours

39. What part of the blood contains the blood group antigen?

    a. Red blood cells
    b. White blood cells
    c. Platelets
    d. Serum
    e. Plasma

40. Which of these is not one of the blood type groups?

    a. AB–
    b. OA+
    c. A–
    d. B–
    e. AB+

41. Which of these statements is accurate regarding blood types?

    a. A person with AB blood has both A and B antibodies.
    b. A person with AB blood has neither the A nor B antigens.
    c. A person in the A blood group has type A antibodies.
    d. A person in the A blood group has type B antigens.
    e. A person with O blood has neither the A nor B antigens.

42. The universal blood donor is blood type:

    a. O negative.
    b. B negative.
    c. A negative.
    d. AB positive.
    e. A positive.

43. The universal recipient of blood is type:

    a. O negative.
    b. B negative.
    c. A negative.
    d. AB positive.
    e. A positive.

44. Which of these represents a critical situation regarding Rh factor?

    a. A pregnant woman who did not receive RhoGAM prior to her first pregnancy
    b. An Rh-negative woman who becomes pregnant with an Rh-positive baby
    c. An Rh-negative woman who becomes pregnant from an Rh-negative father
    d. An Rh-negative pregnant woman carrying an Rh-negative baby in her first pregnancy
    e. An Rh-positive woman who becomes pregnant with an Rh-positive baby

45. Which of these individuals would probably not be able to donate blood?

    a. A person who weighs 125 pounds
    b. A 60-year-old postmenopausal woman
    c. A 14-year-old male
    d. A person with a hemoglobin of 16 g/dL
    e. A person with a blood pressure of 130/82

46. Which type of immunity occurs when a person is exposed to a foreign antigen such as pollen and the body reacts with symptoms?

    a. Active natural immunity
    b. Active induced immunity
    c. Acquired induced immunity
    d. Passive natural immunity
    e. Passive induced immunity

47. What type of immunity exists when antibodies cross from a mother to the fetus through the placenta?

    a. Active natural immunity
    b. Active induced immunity
    c. Acquired induced immunity
    d. Passive natural immunity
    e. Passive induced immunity

48. Which type of immunoglobulin antibody functions in reaction to intestinal worms?

    a. IgA
    b. IgD
    c. IgE
    d. IgG
    e. IgM

49. Which of these tests is not a type of immunology testing?

    a. Hepatitis A and B
    b. Mononucleosis
    c. Pregnancy
    d. Hematocrit
    e. Blood typing

BRIEF EXPLANATIONS

50. Explain the difference between an antigen and an antibody.

_____

_____

_____

_____

51. Describe the function of each of these immunoglobulins.

IgA: _____

IgD: _____

IgE: _____

IgG: _____

IgM: _____

52. Explain how an agglutination test is determined to be either negative or positive.

_____

_____

_____

_____

53. What are three causes of a false-positive or false-negative result when performing agglutination testing?

_____

_____

_____

_____

54. Explain why it is important to follow proper handling and storage of reagents in testing kits. Provide two improper handling methods.

_____

_____

_____

_____

WHAT DO YOU DO?

55. Read the following scenario and respond to the questions with a short answer.

Sonya Taylor is pregnant with her first baby. The physician asked the medical assistant to draw blood for prenatal testing including a test to determine her blood type. The patient asks the medical assistant why it is necessary to find out what her blood type is. She is concerned that it is not normal to perform that test and that the physician suspects a problem with the pregnancy. The physician did not explain the reason for the test.

a. What would you say to this patient to reassure her that this is normal prenatal testing?

_____

_____

_____

_____

b. Her blood test results reveal that she is Rh negative and she knows the father is Rh positive. How would you explain the treatment she needs following the delivery?

_____

_____

_____

_____

PATIENT EDUCATION

56. Write a short narrative script that you can use to provide patient education explaining the benefits of breast-feeding and the effect on the baby's immunity.

_____

_____

_____

_____

INTERNET RESEARCH

Visit the Centers for Disease Control and Prevention Web site at www.cdc.gov and research infectious mononucleosis. According to the information provided at this site, what are the symptoms, methods of transmission, prevention, and treatment of this disease?

_____

_____

_____

_____

_____

_____

_____

Procedure 26-1 | Performing an HCG Pregnancy Test

Name: _____ **Date:** _____ **Time:** _____ **Grade:** _____

Equipment: Pregnancy test kit, timer or clock, patient's specimen, gloves, lab form, patient chart, and control log

Performance Requirement: Student will perform this skill with ____% accuracy not to exceed _____ minutes. (Instructor will determine the point value for each step, % accuracy, and minutes required.)

Performance Checklist

Point Value	Performance Points Earned	Procedure Steps
		1. Wash your hands and apply gloves.
		2. Assemble the test kit's equipment. The kit should be at room temperature.
		3. Check that the names on the specimen container and lab form are the same.
		4. Use one test pack for the patient and one for each control.
		5. Label three test packs as follows: the patient's name, "positive control," and "negative control."
		6. In the patient's chart and the control log, record the type of specimen obtained (urine or plasma/serum).
		7. Use a transfer pipette to aspirate the specimen. Place four drops in the sample well of the test pack labeled with the patient's name.
		8. Carefully aspirate the positive control and place four drops in the sample well of the test pack labeled "positive control."
		9. Carefully aspirate the negative control and place four drops in the sample well of the test pack labeled "negative control."
		10. Set a timer for the amount of time specified by the manufacturer of the test.
		11. Consult the test manufacturer's insert in the kit to interpret test results. The insert will tell you what to look for in reading a positive or negative result.
		12. Report the results when the end-of-assay window is read and after you have checked the controls for accuracy.
		13. Record the controls and patient's information on the work sheet or log form and in the patient's records.
		14. Clean up the work area and dispose of all waste properly. Remove gloves and wash hands.

Procedure 26-1	Performing an HCG Pregnancy Test (*Continued*)

CALCULATION

Total Points Possible: _____

Total Points Earned: _____

Points Earned/Points Possible = _____%

Student completion time (minutes): _____

PASS   FAIL   COMMENTS:

_____

Student's signature _____   Date _____

Instructor's signature _____   Date _____

| Procedure 26-2 | Performing a Group a Rapid Strep Test |

Name: _____ Date: _____ Time: _____ Grade: _____

Equipment: Rapid strep A test kit, patient culture swab, gloves, lab form, and the patient's medical record.

Performance Requirement: Student will perform this skill with ____% accuracy not to exceed _____ minutes. (Instructor will determine the point value for each step, % accuracy, and minutes required.)

Performance Checklist

Point Value	Performance Points Earned	Procedure Steps
		1. Wash your hands and apply gloves.
		2. Check that the names on the specimen container and the lab form are the same.
		3. Label one extraction tube with the patient's name, one with "positive control," and one with "negative control."
		4. Follow the kit directions. Carefully add the correct reagents and drops to each of the extraction tubes.
		5. Insert the patient's culture swab into the labeled extraction tube.
		6. Add the correct controls to each of the two control tubes and place a sterile swab into each control tube.
		7. Use the swab to mix each tube's contents by twirling each swab five to six times.
		8. Set a timer for the time specified by the manufacturer of the test.
		9. Draw the swab up from the bottom of each tube and out of any liquid. Press out all fluid on the swab head by rolling the swab against the inside of the tube before it is withdrawn.
		10. Add three drops from the well-mixed extraction tube to the sample window of the strep A test unit labeled with the patient's name. Do the same for each control.
		11. Set the timer for the correct amount of time.
		12. A positive result will show up as a line in the result window within 5 minutes.
		13. A negative result is indicated if no line appears within 5 minutes. However, you must wait exactly 5 minutes to read a negative result, to avoid getting a false negative.
		14. Verify the control results before recording any test results. Log the controls and the patient's information into your log or work sheet.
		15. Clean up the work area and dispose of all waste in the right place.
		16. Remove gloves and wash hands.

Procedure 26-2 | Performing a Group a Rapid Strep Test (*Continued*)

CALCULATION

Total Points Possible: _____

Total Points Earned: _____

Points Earned/Points Possible = _____ %

Student completion time (minutes): _____

PASS   FAIL   COMMENTS:

_____

Student's signature _____   Date _____

Instructor's signature _____   Date _____

Chapter Objectives

- Explain why urinalysis is performed and the role of the medical assistant in this procedure.
- Describe the methods of urine collection.
- Perform a physical analysis of a urine specimen.
- Perform a chemical reagent test strip analysis.
- Explain the purpose of a urine culture.
- Identify the physical properties of urine and cite various conditions that can affect them.
- List the main chemical substances that may be found in urine and their significance.
- Prepare urine specimen for microscopic examination.
- Identify substances that might be present in urine sediment.
- Describe the process of microscopic examination of urine sediment.
- Describe how urine pregnancy tests are conducted.
- Describe how urine drug testing is conducted.

CAAHEP & ABHES Competencies

CAAHEP

- Obtain specimens and perform CLIA-waived urinalysis.
- Identify CLIA-waived tests associated with common diseases.
- Differentiate between normal and abnormal test results.

ABHES

- Perform selected CLIA-waived tests that assist with diagnosis and treatment.
- Perform urinalysis.
- Perform kit testing for pregnancy.
- Collect, label, and process specimens.
- Instruct patients in the collection of clean-catch midstream urine specimen.
- Instruct patient in the collection of a 24-hour urine specimen.
- Practice quality control.

TERMINOLOGY MATCHING

Directions: Match the terms in Column A with the definitions in Column B.

Column A

1. _____ Bacteriuria
2. _____ Casts
3. _____ Catheter
4. _____ Culture
5. _____ Diuretics
6. _____ Glycosuria
7. _____ Hematuria
8. _____ Hyperglycemia
9. _____ Ketones
10. _____ Myoglobin
11. _____ Postprandial
12. _____ Pyuria
13. _____ Random urine
14. _____ Specific gravity
15. _____ Turbid

Column B

a. Pus in the urine indicating possible infection in the bladder or kidneys
b. Sugar or glucose in the urine that usually indicates diabetes mellitus
c. Bacteria in urine
d. Blood in the urine that usually indicates injury or disease in the urinary system
e. After eating a meal
f. Drugs that increase the body's fluid output resulting in more urine production
g. High blood sugar
h. Cylinders of proteins and other substances that form and solidify in the nephron tubules in the kidneys
i. Chemicals the body makes when it metabolizes (breaks down) fat
j. A thin sterile, flexible tube inserted into the bladder through the urethra to drain the bladder of urine
k. A red protein containing heme that carries and stores oxygen in muscle cells
l. Colonies of bacteria grown under controlled conditions in a container in a lab
m. Comparing the consistency of a substance compared to the weight of water
n. Used to describe cloudy urine; probably contains particulate matter or tiny solid particles
o. Urine specimen collected at anytime

DEFINING ABBREVIATIONS

Directions: Provide the specific meaning of each of the following abbreviations. Watch your spelling.

16. C&S: _____

_____

17. HCG: _____

_____

18. pH: _____

_____

19. POL: _____

_____

20. PPM: _____

_____

21. UTI: _____

_____

MAKING IT RIGHT

Each of the following statements is false. Rewrite the statement to make it a true statement.

22. A random urine is a test in which bacteria and other microbes are grown in a lab.

_____

_____

_____

_____

23. Urine specimens should be tested within 3 to 4 hours after collection because the specimen will begin deteriorating after that time.

_____

_____

_____

_____

24. Fluorescein in the urine, as in jaundice, may indicate possible liver disease including hepatitis.

_____

_____

_____

_____

25. Urine that is clear probably contains particulate matter, tiny solid particles, or white blood cells.

_____

_____

_____

_____

26. When performing a specific gravity, dilute urine will have a higher specific gravity.

_____

_____

_____

_____

27. A patient should submit a urine specimen when fasting, nothing to eat or drink for 12 to 16 hours.

_____

_____

_____

_____

28. Urobilinogen is a chemical the body makes when it metabolizes (breaks down) fat.

_____

_____

_____

_____

MULTIPLE CHOICE

Directions: Choose the best answer for each question.

29. Which of these would show positive on chemical testing if there is a large amount of bacteria in the urine?

   a. Bilirubin
   b. Ketone
   c. Urobilinogen
   d. Nitrite
   e. Glucose

30. A confirmation test for ketones in the urine is:

   a. Acetest.
   b. Ictotest.
   c. Clinitest.
   d. sulfosalicylic acid test.
   e. bilirubin test.

31. What does CLIA require to perform microscopic exam of urine sediment?

   a. Waived status
   b. POL accreditation
   c. PPM certificate
   d. Certified medical assistant
   e. CMS accreditation

32. Which of these is not identified in a microscopic urinalysis?

   a. White blood cells
   b. Red blood cells
   c. Waxy casts
   d. Epithelial cells
   e. Glucose crystals

33. Myoglobin in the urine may cause a positive reading on the chemical test.

   a. Glucose
   b. Blood
   c. Nitrite
   d. pH
   e. Ketone

34. What drug is not one of those employers consider a concern if found in urine?

   a. Opiates
   b. Methadone
   c. Cocaine
   d. Penicillin
   e. Marijuana

35. If a physician wants to evaluate a patient's ability to metabolize glucose after eating, what type of urine test is ordered?

   a. Random
   b. 24-hour
   c. Postprandial
   d. Midstream clean catch
   e. Catheterized

36. What is the primary reason for collecting a midstream clean-catch urine specimen?

    a. It eliminates most contamination from the patient's skin.
    b. It is easiest for the patient to collect.
    c. It will guarantee a fresh specimen.
    d. It will remove all bacteria from the urine.
    e. It provides a cleaner specimen than other methods.

37. Which of these statements is not true regarding the collection of a specimen for a urine culture?

    a. A sterile container is used to collect the specimen.
    b. There is no time requirement for the specimen collection.
    c. The patient must wear sterile gloves when collecting the specimen.
    d. The specimen collection does not require the patient to be fasting.
    e. The medical assistant must wear sterile gloves to handle the specimen container.

38. Which of these urine collection methods is performed by the physician?

    a. 2-hour postprandial
    b. Midstream clean catch
    c. 24-hour collection
    d. Bladder catheterization
    e. Suprapubic aspiration

39. Which of these is a critical instruction for a patient collecting a 24-hour urine?

    a. Restrict fluid intake during the 24-hour period.
    b. Refrigerate the container during the collection time.
    c. Collect urine only during daytime hours.
    d. Do not take routine medications until all collection is completed.
    e. Do no drink any beverages with caffeine since this will increase your urine output.

40. What is the normal range for specific gravity of urine?

    a. 1.000 to 1.003
    b. 1.003 to 1.035
    c. 1.020 to 1.040
    d. 1.025 to 1.050
    e. 1.030 to 1.060

41. What change will start to take place in urine if not tested within 1 hour of collection?

    a. The pH will change from alkaline to acid.
    b. Cloudy urine will become clearer.
    c. Microorganisms will die and the urine will not accurately test for bacteria.
    d. The glucose level will become lower due to bacteria consuming it as a nutrient.
    e. The specific gravity will become lower indicating it is more like the specific gravity of water.

42. Which of these drugs are prescribed to increase the body's fluid output resulting in more urine production?

    a. Antihypertensives
    b. Analgesics
    c. Bronchodilators
    d. Antihistamines
    e. Diuretics

43. Which of these substances in the urine would not cause turbid urine?

    a. Epithelial cells
    b. Pus
    c. Acidic pH
    d. Red blood cells
    e. Bacteria

44. Specific gravity is a comparison of the weight of urine and the weight of:

    a. plasma.
    b. serum.
    c. lymph fluid.
    d. water.
    e. blood.

45. A urine that has a strong ammonia odor will usually have a high level of:

    a. bacteria.
    b. ketones.
    c. protein.
    d. red blood cells.
    e. glucose.

46. What is the expected normal range or result for ketones in the urine?

    a. Negative
    b. Positive
    c. 6.0
    d. 1.010
    e. Moderate

47. What pH reading represents a neutral level, not acid or alkaline?

    a. 5.5
    b. 6.0
    c. 6.5
    d. 7.0
    e. 8.0

48. Which of these terms means glucose in urine?

    a. Hyperglycemia
    b. Glucosuria
    c. Hypoglycemia
    d. Glycemia
    e. Polyuria

49. A Clinitest is used to confirm the presence of:

    a. fat.
    b. protein.
    c. glucose.
    d. blood.
    e. bacteria.

50. The substance found in urine when there is a breakdown of fat is:

    a. cholesterol.
    b. glucose.
    c. protein.
    d. nitrite.
    e. ketone.

51. What substance is positive in the urine due to a breakdown of hemoglobin?

    a. Nitrite
    b. Bilirubin
    c. Protein
    d. Ketone
    e. Glucose

52. Which of these would cause a positive nitrite reading?

    a. Glucosuria
    b. Hematuria
    c. Bacteriuria
    d. Ketonuria
    e. Proteinuria

53. A cast in the urine forms in the:

    a. bladder.
    b. urethra.
    c. ureter.
    d. kidney.
    e. urethral meatus.

BRIEF EXPLANATIONS

54. Explain the significance of these types of epithelial cells in the urine.

    a. Squamous epithelial cells: _____

    b. Transitional epithelial cells: _____

    c. Renal epithelial cells: _____

55. Explain why the physician orders these types of urine specimens.

    a. Random: _____

    b. Postprandial: _____

    c. 24-hour: _____

56. Explain why a first morning urine specimen is preferred for urine pregnancy testing.

    _____
    _____
    _____
    _____

57. Explain why the physician would order a urine culture and sensitivity.

_____

_____

_____

_____

58. Why is it important to refrigerate urine if not able to test within 1 hour of collection? What changes can take place?

_____

_____

_____

_____

WHAT DO YOU DO?

59. Read the following scenario and respond to the questions with a short answer.

Paula Thomas is a 17-year-old patient who is having burning and pain with urination. She states that she has never had this problem before. The medical assistant instructs her to collect midstream clean-catch urine for testing. As she delivers the urine specimen to the medical assistant, the patient asks what might be wrong with her and is it serious.

a. How would you respond to the patient's questions?

_____

_____

_____

_____

b. The patient's urinalysis reveals a significant urinary tract infection. He orders a culture and sensitivity. How will you have the patient collect the specimen for this test?

_____

_____

_____

_____

c. How would you explain to the patient the need to have a C&S performed?

_____

_____

_____

_____

PATIENT EDUCATION

60. Write a short narrative script that you can use to provide patient education about the need for proper hydration. Explain how dehydration can affect the function of the kidneys.

_____

_____

_____

_____

INTERNET RESEARCH

Visit the National Institutes for Health Web site at www.nih.gov and research cystitis. What are causes and risk factors to develop UTI? What are ways to avoid developing UTI?

_____

_____

_____

_____

_____

_____

_____

| Procedure 27-1 | Obtaining a Clean-Catch Midstream Urine Specimen | |

Name: _____   Date: _____   Time: _____   Grade: _____

Equipment: Clean, dry (or sterile) urine container labeled with the patient's name, antiseptic wipes, and gloves

Performance Requirement: Student will perform this skill with ____% accuracy not to exceed _____ minutes. (Instructor will determine the point value for each step, % accuracy, and minutes required.)

Performance Checklist

Point Value	Performance Points Earned	Procedure Steps
		1. Wash your hands and put on gloves if you are assisting the patient.
		2. Greet and identify the patient. Explain the procedure and give the patient the collection container and antiseptic wipes.
		3. Provide cleansing instructions for male or female patient.
		4. Instruct patient to wash hands before and after collection.
		5. Explain proper handling of the container without contaminating it or the lid.
		6. Explain proper collection of midstream specimen.
		7. Use gloves when handling the specimen container returned by the patient.
		8. Clean the work area, remove your gloves, and wash your hands.
		9. Test, transfer, or store the container according to the office policy.
		10. Document the procedure in the patient's medical record.

CALCULATION

Total Points Possible: _____

Total Points Earned: _____

Points Earned/Points Possible = _____%

Student completion time (minutes): _____

PASS   FAIL   COMMENTS:

_____

Student's signature _____   Date _____

Instructor's signature _____   Date _____

Procedure 27-2 | Determining Color and Clarity of Urine

Name: _____ Date: _____ Time: _____ Grade: _____

Equipment: Clear test tube, a sheet of white paper with scored black lines, and a patient report form or data form, and gloves

Performance Requirement: Student will perform this skill with ____% accuracy not to exceed _____ minutes. (Instructor will determine the point value for each step, % accuracy, and minutes required.)

Performance Checklist

Point Value	Performance Points Earned	Procedure Steps
		1. Wash your hands and put on gloves. Apply other PPE if required by office policy (gown, face shield).
		2. Verify that the patient name on the specimen container and the report form are the same.
		3. Pour 10 to 15 mL of urine from the container into the test tube.
		4. In a bright light against a white background, examine the color of the urine in the tube.
		5. Determine urine clarity by holding the tube in front of the white paper scored with black lines. Record as clear, hazy, cloudy, or turbid.
		6. If further testing is required but will be delayed more than an hour, refrigerate the specimen to avoid chemical changes.
		7. Properly care for or dispose of equipment and supplies. Clean the work area using a 10% bleach solution.
		8. Remove your gloves and other PPE if used. Wash your hands.
		9. Record the results of the physical findings.

CALCULATION

Total Points Possible: _____

Total Points Earned: _____

Points Earned/Points Possible = _____%

Student completion time (minutes): _____

PASS   FAIL   COMMENTS:

_____

Student's signature _____ Date _____

Instructor's signature _____ Date _____

Procedure 27-3   Performing a Chemical Reagent Strip Analysis

Name: _____ Date: _____ Time: _____ Grade: _____

Equipment: Chemical strip (Multistix or Chemstrip), the manufacturer's color comparison chart, a stopwatch or timer, a 15- × 125-mm test tube or KOVA system urine tube, paper towel (absorbent disposable towel), patient report form or data form, and gloves

Performance Requirement: Student will perform this skill with _____% accuracy not to exceed _____ minutes. (Instructor will determine the point value for each step, % accuracy, and minutes required.)

Performance Checklist

Point Value	Performance Points Earned	Procedure Steps
		1. Wash your hands and apply gloves. Apply other PPE if required by office policy.
		2. Verify that the names on the specimen container and the report form are the same.
		3. Mix the patient's urine by gently swirling the specimen container. Then, pour 12 mL of urine into a KOVA system urine tube.
		4. Remove a reagent strip from its container and replace the lid to prevent deterioration of the strips by humidity.
		5. Immerse the reagent strip in the urine completely and then immediately remove it, sliding the edge of the strip along the lip of the tube to remove excess urine. Turn the strip on its edge and touch the edge to a paper towel or other absorbent paper.
		6. Start your stopwatch or timer immediately after removing the strip from the urine. Reactions must be read at specific times as directed in the package insert and on the color comparison chart.
		7. Compare the reagent pads to the color chart.
		8. Read all the reactions at the times indicated and record the results.
		9. Discard the used strip in a biohazard container. Discard the urine in accordance with the office policies.
		10. Properly care for or dispose of equipment and supplies. Clean the work area using a 10% bleach solution.
		11. Remove PPE and wash your hands.

| Procedure 27-3 | Performing a Chemical Reagent Strip Analysis (*Continued*) |

CALCULATION

Total Points Possible: _____

Total Points Earned: _____

Points Earned/Points Possible = _____%

Student completion time (minutes): _____

PASS   FAIL   COMMENTS:

_____

Student's signature _____ Date _____

Instructor's signature _____ Date _____

Procedure 27-4 | Preparing Urine Sediment for Microscopic Examination

Name: _____ **Date:** _____ **Time:** _____ **Grade:** _____

Equipment: Centrifuge, urine centrifuge tubes, a transfer pipette, microscope slide, coverslip, a patient report form or data form, and gloves (Sedi-Stain if required by office policy)

Performance Requirement: Student will perform this skill with _____% accuracy not to exceed _____ minutes. (Instructor will determine the point value for each step, % accuracy, and minutes required.)

Performance Checklist

Point Value	Performance Points Earned	Procedure Steps
		1. Wash your hands and gather supplies.
		2. Verify that the names on the specimen container and the report form are the same.
		3. Swirl the specimen to mix. Pour 10 or 12 mL of well-mixed urine into a labeled urine centrifuge tube or a tube provided by the test system manufacturer. Cap the tube with a plastic cap.
		4. Centrifuge the sample at 1,500 rpm for 5 minutes. If only one urine tube, use a counterweighted tube filled with water.
		5. When the centrifuge has stopped, remove the tubes. Pour off all but 0.5 to 1.0 mL of the fluid.
		6. Suspend the sediment again in the remaining supernatant by aspirating up into the bulbous portion of a urine transfer pipette.
		7. If sediment stain used, put appropriate number of drops in the urine tube.
		8. Place a microscope slide (KOVA slide or other urine system slide) on the counter. Add a drop of the mixed sediment on the slide and place a coverslip over the drop.
		9. The slide is now prepared for review by a qualified person. Medical assistant is not qualified.
		10. Properly care for or dispose of equipment and supplies. Clean the work area using a 10%bleach solution.
		11. Remove your PPE. Wash your hands.

| Procedure 27-4 | Preparing Urine Sediment for Microscopic Examination (*Continued*) |

CALCULATION

Total Points Possible: _____

Total Points Earned: _____

Points Earned/Points Possible = _____%

Student completion time (minutes): _____

PASS   FAIL   COMMENTS:

_____

Student's signature _____ Date _____

Instructor's signature _____ Date _____

Procedure 27-5 | Urine Collection from Infants

Name: _____ Date: _____ Time: _____ Grade: _____

Equipment: Gloves, personal antiseptic wipes, pediatric urine collection bag, completed laboratory request slip, and biohazard transport container

Performance Requirement: Student will perform this skill with _____% accuracy not to exceed _____ minutes. (Instructor will determine the point value for each step, % accuracy, and minutes required.)

Performance Checklist

Point Value	Performance Points Earned	Procedure Steps
		1. Wash your hands and gather supplies.
		2. Explain the procedure to the parents.
		3. Place the infant in a lying position on their back. Ask for help from parents as needed.
		4. After putting on gloves, clean the genitalia with the antiseptic wipes. Use proper technique for female and male infants.
		5. Holding the collection device, remove the upper portion of the paper backing and press it around the mons pubis.
		6. Remove the second section and press it against the perineum. Loosely attach a diaper.
		7. Give the infant fluids, unless otherwise indicated. Check the collection device frequently.
		8. When the infant has voided, remove the collection device and diaper.
		9. Clean the skin of any adhesive that remains.
		10. Prepare the specimen for transport to the laboratory or process it according to office policy.
		11. Remove your gloves and wash your hands.
		12. Record the procedure in the patient's chart.

Procedure 27-5 | Urine Collection from Infants (*Continued*)

CALCULATION

Total Points Possible: _____

Total Points Earned: _____

Points Earned/Points Possible = _____%

Student completion time (minutes): _____

PASS   FAIL   COMMENTS:

_____

Student's signature _____   Date _____

Instructor's signature _____   Date _____

Chapter Objectives

- Explain the purpose of performing clinical chemistry tests.
- List the common panels of chemistry tests.
- List the instruments used for chemical testing.
- List tests used to evaluate renal function.
- List the common electrolytes and explain the relationship of electrolytes to body function.
- Describe the nonprotein nitrogenous compounds and name conditions associated with abnormal values.
- Describe the substances commonly tested in liver function assessment.
- Explain thyroid function and identify the hormone that regulates the thyroid gland.
- Describe how laboratory tests help assess for a myocardial infarction.
- Describe how pancreatitis is diagnosed with laboratory tests.
- Explain how the body uses and regulates glucose and summarize the purpose of the major glucose tests.
- Determine a patient's blood glucose level.
- Perform glucose tolerance testing.
- Describe the function of cholesterol and other lipids and their correlation to heart disease.

CAAHEP & ABHES Competencies

CAAHEP

- Perform patient screening using established protocols.
- Obtain specimens and perform CLIA-waived chemistry tests.
- Differentiate between normal and abnormal test results.
- Reassure a patient of the accuracy of the test results.

ABHES

- Practice quality control.
- Perform selected CLIA-waived chemistry tests that assist with diagnosis and treatment.
- Collect, label, and process specimens.

TERMINOLOGY MATCHING

Directions: Match the terms in Column A with the definitions in Column B.

Column A

1. _____ Bilirubin
2. _____ Electrolytes
3. _____ Hyperkalemia
4. _____ Hypernatremia
5. _____ Hyperuricemia
6. _____ Hypocalcemia
7. _____ Hypochloremia
8. _____ Hypoglycemia
9. _____ Hypokalemia
10. _____ Hyponatremia
11. _____ Nitrogenous

Column B

a. Ions in blood and body fluids, chemicals that carry an electrical charge
b. Low blood sugar
c. Relating to, or containing, nitrogen
d. Uric acid levels above the normal range
e. Serum potassium level below the normal level of 3.5 mEq/L
f. Amber-colored substance produced as a by-product of hemoglobin breakdown
g. Sodium levels above the normal 145 mEq/L level
h. Sodium levels below 135 mEq/L
i. Potassium level is above 5.0 mEq/L
j. Serum chloride level that drops below 96 mEq/L
k. Calcium levels below the normal level of 8.5 mg/dL

DEFINING ABBREVIATIONS

Directions: Provide the specific meaning of each of the following abbreviations. Watch your spelling.

12. ALT: _____

_____

13. ALP: _____

_____

14. AST: _____

_____

15. BUN: _____

_____

16. CK: _____

_____

17. CMP: _____

_____

18. FBS: _____

_____

19. GTT: _____

_____

20. HbA1C: _____

_____

21. HCO_3: _____

_____

22. HDL: _____

_____

23. LDL: _____

_____

24. POL: _____

_____

25. PP: _____

_____

26. TSH: _____

_____

MAKING IT RIGHT

Each of the following statements is false. Rewrite the statement to make it a true statement.

27. Knowing the level of bilirubin in a patient's blood helps show how well the patient's pancreas is functioning.

_____

_____

_____

_____

28. The gallbladder rids the body of waste products and helps maintain fluid balance and acid–base balance.

_____

_____

_____

_____

29. Hypochloremia occurs from acute or chronic renal failure or electrolyte imbalance due to hypoparathyroidism, underactive parathyroid glands.

_____

_____

_____

_____

30. If bicarbonate levels are increased, the patient develops acidosis, a condition when the pH is too basic.

_____

_____

_____

_____

31. Urea causes many newborns to appear jaundiced or yellow, a few days after birth.

_____

_____

_____

_____

32. Amylase and lipase are two endocrine system products of the pancreas.

_____

_____

_____

_____

33. Calcium, an important hormone, transports the glucose into the body's cells.

_____

_____

_____

_____

MULTIPLE CHOICE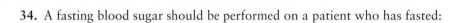

Directions: Choose the best answer for each question.

34. A fasting blood sugar should be performed on a patient who has fasted:

   a. 2 to 4 hours.
   b. 4 to 8 hours.
   c. 8 to 12 hours.
   d. 12 to 16 hours.
   e. 18 to 24 hours.

35. The normal HbA1C is less than:

   a. 2.5%.
   b. 3.5%.
   c. 4.5%.
   d. 6.5%.
   e. 8.0%.

36. The American Heart Association recommends that the cholesterol level in the blood be less than:

   a. 100 mg/dL.
   b. 150 mg/dL.
   c. 200 mg/dL.
   d. 275 mg/dL.
   e. 300 mg/dL.

37. In order for a medical assistant to perform chemistry tests in the office, the test must be:

    a. able to complete within 5 minutes.
    b. ordered by the physician.
    c. inexpensive.
    d. able to complete from a capillary specimen.
    e. CLIA waived.

38. Which of these instruments measures light in a solution to determine the concentration of substances?

    a. Centrifuge
    b. Spectrophotometer
    c. Incubator
    d. Sphygmomanometer
    e. Hemocytometer

39. Ions in blood and body fluids are:

    a. electrolytes.
    b. hormones.
    c. serum and plasma.
    d. red and white blood cells.
    e. lipids.

40. What condition occurs when a patient's sodium level is above 145 mEq/L?

    a. Hypercalcemia
    b. Hypocalcemia
    c. Hypernatremia
    d. Hyponatremia
    e. Hyperkalemia

41. Hypoparathyroidism can cause a significantly low level of blood:

    a. cholesterol.
    b. glucose.
    c. insulin.
    d. calcium.
    e. chloride.

42. Which of these plays a major role in the delicate acid–base balance and occurs when carbon dioxide dissolves in the bloodstream?

    a. BUN
    b. HCO_3
    c. H_2O
    d. CO_2
    e. HDL

43. A BUN test evaluates the function of the:

    a. kidneys.
    b. heart.
    c. gallbladder.
    d. pancreas.
    e. liver.

44. Which of these is not an electrolyte?

    a. Sodium
    b. Calcium
    c. Potassium
    d. Chloride
    e. Urea

45. Muscle weakness and cramping is commonly caused from low blood:

    a. nitrogen.
    b. albumin.
    c. chloride.
    d. potassium.
    e. magnesium.

46. The normal pH of blood is:

    a. 6.20 to 6.50.
    b. 7.15 to 7.25.
    c. 7.35 to 7.45.
    d. 7.60 to 8.0.
    e. 8.0 to 8.25.

47. Urea is a waste product that forms in the:

    a. liver.
    b. heart.
    c. kidneys.
    d. pancreas.
    e. intestines.

48. Which of these substances is a by-product of protein metabolism?

    a. Bicarbonate
    b. Uric acid
    c. Calcium
    d. Potassium
    e. Sodium

49. Which of these substances is a by-product of hemoglobin breakdown?

    a. Albumin
    b. Creatine kinase
    c. Bilirubin
    d. Uric acid
    e. Amylase

50. A primary source of energy for the body is:

    a. lipase.
    b. amylase.
    c. albumin.
    d. nitrogen.
    e. glucose.

51. What enzyme is released into the bloodstream when a patient experiences a myocardial infarction?

a. HDL
b. ALT
c. BUN
d. CK
e. AST

52. Which of these is not included in a lipid profile?

a. Total cholesterol
b. Triglyceride
c. Fasting glucose
d. HDL
e. LDL

53. To confirm a diagnosis of gestational diabetes, the physician would order a:

a. HDL.
b. LDL.
c. TSH.
d. GTT.
e. BUN.

54. Hypokalemia is a condition of a low blood:

a. potassium.
b. calcium.
c. chloride.
d. sodium.
e. magnesium.

55. Which of these statements best describes alkalosis?

a. A condition caused from a lack of bicarbonate.
b. A condition when the pH is too basic.
c. A condition when the pH is to acidic.
d. It is a waste product of hemoglobin breakdown.
e. It is a by-product of protein metabolism in the blood.

56. Gout is commonly caused from:

a. hyperchloremia.
b. hypoglycemia.
c. hyperkalemia.
d. hypocalcemia.
e. hyperuricemia.

57. ALP, ALT, and AST are tests performed to evaluate:

a. pancreas function.
b. kidney function.
c. heart function.
d. liver function.
e. thyroid function.

58. Which symptom is most common when there is an elevated bilirubin in the blood?

   a. Malnutrition
   b. Dehydration
   c. Jaundice
   d. Muscle cramps
   e. Fatigue

BRIEF EXPLANATIONS

59. List four body fluids used to perform chemistry tests.

   _____

   _____

   _____

   _____

60. Explain why it is important for the medical assistant to understand the purpose of chemistry tests and what abnormal results may mean for the patient.

   _____

   _____

   _____

   _____

61. Why is it important for the body to maintain acid–base balance? Provide an example of what can happen if this balance is not maintained.

   _____

   _____

   _____

   _____

62. Why would a physician order a lipid panel?

   _____

   _____

   _____

   _____

63. Provide three (3) conditions or symptoms that are caused by a potassium level that is too high or too low.

   _____

   _____

   _____

   _____

WHAT DO YOU DO?

64. Read the following scenario and respond to the questions with a short answer.

Elizabeth Baker is a 28-year-old patient who is in the second trimester of her pregnancy. She is experiencing symptoms including excessive thirst and frequent urination. The physician orders a glucose tolerance test. The medical assistant is providing instructions and setting the appointment for the patient. The patient starts crying stating that she is scared that there might be something wrong with the baby.

a. What would you say to try to reassure this patient?

_____

_____

_____

_____

b. What does the patient need to do to prepare for the GTT?

_____

_____

_____

_____

c. What condition is the physician suspecting with this patient?

_____

_____

_____

_____

PATIENT EDUCATION

65. Write a short narrative script that you can use to provide patient education of how lipids in the blood can affect the condition of the heart and circulatory system.

_____

_____

_____

_____

INTERNET RESEARCH

Visit the WebMD Web site at www.webmd.com and research the condition metabolic syndrome. What is it? What are treatments for it and how can it be prevented?

_____

_____

_____

_____

_____

_____

_____

_____

| Procedure 28-1 | Determining Blood Glucose | |

Name: _____ Date: _____ Time: _____ Grade: _____

Equipment: Glucose meter, glucose reagent strips, a lancet, an alcohol pad, sterile gauze, a paper towel, an adhesive bandage, and gloves.

Performance Requirement: Student will perform this skill with ____% accuracy not to exceed _____ minutes. (Instructor will determine the point value for each step, % accuracy, and minutes required.)

Performance Checklist

Point Value	Performance Points Earned	Procedure Steps
		1. Wash your hands and put on your gloves before you remove the reagent strip from the container.
		2. Turn on the glucose meter and make sure that it's calibrated correctly.
		3. Remove one reagent strip, lay it on the paper towel, and recap the container. The strip is ready for testing and the paper towel serves as a disposable work surface. It will also absorb any excess blood.
		4. Greet and identify the patient. Explain the procedure. Ask the patient when they last ate and document this in her chart.
		5. Cleanse the puncture site (finger) with alcohol.
		6. Perform a capillary puncture. Wipe away the first drop of blood.
		7. Turn the patient's hand palm down and gently squeeze the finger so that a large drop of blood forms.
		8. Bring the reagent strip up to the finger and touch the strip to the blood. Make sure you do not touch the finger.
		9. Insert the reagent strip into the glucose meter. Some devices require that the strip is inserted prior to applying the drop of blood.
		10. Apply pressure to the puncture wound with gauze.
		11. The instrument reads the reaction strip and displays the result on the screen in milligrams per deciliter (mg/dL).
		12. Apply a small adhesive bandage to the patient's fingertip.
		13. Properly dispose the equipment and supplies. Clean the work area. Remove your gloves and wash your hands.
		14. Document the procedure and results in the patient's medical record.

(Continued)

Procedure 28-1   Determining Blood Glucose (*Continued*)

CALCULATION

Total Points Possible: _____

Total Points Earned: _____

Points Earned/Points Possible = _____%

Student completion time (minutes): _____

PASS   FAIL   COMMENTS:

_____

Student's signature _____   Date _____

Instructor's signature _____   Date _____

Procedure 28-2 | Glucose Tolerance Testing

Name: _____ Date: _____ Time: _____ Grade: _____

Equipment: Calibrated amount of glucose solution per physician's order, glucose meter equipment, phlebotomy equipment, glucose test strips, alcohol wipes, a stopwatch (timer), and gloves.

Performance Requirement: Student will perform this skill with ____% accuracy not to exceed _____ minutes. (Instructor will determine the point value for each step, % accuracy, and minutes required).

Performance Checklist

Point Value	Performance Points Earned	Procedure Steps
		1. Greet and identify the patient. Explain the procedure, and ask for and answer any questions the patient might have. Ask the patient when he last ate and document this in his chart.
		2. Wash your hands and put on your gloves.
		3. Obtain a fasting glucose (FBS) specimen from the patient by venipuncture or capillary puncture.
		4. If the FBS exceeds 140 mg/dL, do not proceed with the GTT. Inform the physician. If glucose within acceptable range, proceed with the GTT.
		5. Give the glucose drink to the patient and ask the patient to drink it all within 5 minutes.
		6. Note the time the patient finishes the drink; this is the official start of the test.
		7. Obtain another blood specimen exactly 30 minutes after the patient finishes the glucose drink. Label the specimen with the patient's name and time of collection.
		8. The physician may want urine glucose tests done with each blood sample taken.
		9. If the patient does not provide a urine sample, submit an empty urine cup in place and label "patient could not provide urine sample at _____ [time]."
		10. Exactly 1 hour after the glucose drink, obtain another blood and urine specimen.
		11. Exactly 2 hours after the glucose drink, obtain another blood and urine specimen.
		12. Exactly 3 hours after the glucose drink, obtain another blood and urine specimen.
		13. If 3-hour GTT is ordered, the test is now complete; however, it extends by the number of hours the physician ordered (up to 6 hours)

(Continued)

Procedure 28-2 | Glucose Tolerance Testing (*Continued*)

Performance Checklist

Point Value	Performance Points Earned	Procedure Steps
		14. If the specimens are tested by an outside laboratory, package them carefully and arrange for transportation.
		15. Ensure the patient is feeling well and can be released.
		16. Care for and dispose of your equipment and supplies. Clean your work area. Remove your gloves and wash your hands.

CALCULATION

Total Points Possible: _____

Total Points Earned: _____

Points Earned/Points Possible = _____%

Student completion time (minutes): _____

PASS   FAIL   COMMENTS:

_____

Student's signature _____ Date _____

Instructor's signature _____ Date _____

29 Microbiology

Chapter Objectives

- Describe how cultures are used in medical microbiology.
- Name and describe the different types of bacteria.
- Identify the main types of fungi that may be found in the human body.
- Identify different types of viruses.
- Identify the two main types of Metazoa and give at least one example of each.
- Summarize the medical assistant's responsibilities in microbiological testing.
- List the most common microbiological specimens collected in the physician's office lab.
- Collect a specimen for throat culture.
- Collect a sputum specimen.
- Collect a stool specimen.
- Test a stool specimen for occult blood.
- Explain how to transport a specimen.
- State the difference between primary cultures, secondary cultures, and pure cultures.
- Name at least three kinds of media used in cultures.
- Describe how microscopic examination is used in medical microbiology.
- Prepare a wet mount slide.
- State the purpose of Gram staining.

CAAHEP & ABHES Competencies

CAAHEP

- Obtain specimens and perform CLIA-waived microbiology test.
- Differentiate between normal and abnormal test results.

ABHES

- Practice quality control.
- Perform selected CLIA-waived tests that assist with diagnosis and treatment in microbiology testing.
- Collect, label, and process specimens.

TERMINOLOGY MATCHING

Directions: Match the terms in Column A with the definitions in Column B.

Column A

1. _____ Aerobic

2. _____ Anaerobic
3. _____ Bacteriology

4. _____ Colony
5. _____ Colony count

6. _____ Culture
7. _____ Gram negative

8. _____ Gram positive
9. _____ Mycology
10. _____ Normal flora
11. _____ Pathogen
12. _____ Petri dish
13. _____ Spores

14. _____ Sputum

15. _____ Wet mount

Column B

a. An empty glass or plastic container used to hold a solid culture medium, such as blood agar
b. A type of bacteria that stain red with safranin dye
c. Microbes that live in and on the human body without causing any problems or disease, nonpathogenic
d. Requiring oxygen for growth
e. A group of identical bacteria that grow in a culture from one "parent" bacteria
f. Disease-causing microorganisms
g. Measures the amount of bacteria growing in one milliliter of urine or quantity of specimen
h. The science and study of fungi
i. Does not require oxygen for growth
j. Mucus from a patient's lungs; used to prepare a culture
k. A type of bacteria that stain purple with crystal violet dye
l. Microscopic exam of bacteria freely moving in fluid
m. Colonies of bacteria grown under controlled conditions in a container in a lab
n. A form of bacteria that can resist the destructive forces of heat, drying, or chemicals
o. The science and study of bacteria

DEFINING ABBREVIATIONS

Directions: Provide the specific meaning of each of the following abbreviations. Watch your spelling.

16. C&S: _____

_____

17. HAI: _____

_____

18. KOH: _____

_____

19. O&P: _____

_____

MAKING IT RIGHT

Each of the following statements is false. Rewrite the statement to make it a true statement.

20. Microorganisms that can cause disease are normal flora.

_____

_____

_____

_____

21. Cultures are grown in culture media with the help of an autoclave.

_____

_____

_____

_____

22. Tetanus is a very serious form of food poisoning.

_____

_____

_____

_____

23. Bacilli are carried by a particular kind of tick, louse, or mite and can cause Rocky Mountain spotted fever.

_____

_____

_____

_____

24. A spirilla is a bacterium that forms a capsule around itself to protect them from destruction.

_____

_____

_____

_____

25. Diseases caused by cocci are mycotic infections, or mycoses.

_____

_____

_____

_____

26. Viruses are single-celled parasitic animals that may be diagnosed in the parasitology laboratory.

_____

_____

_____

_____

MULTIPLE CHOICE

Directions: Choose the best answer for each question.

27. Mites, lice, ticks, and fleas belong to the group of organisms called:

    a. spirochetes.
    b. Protozoa.
    c. Rickettsias.
    d. arthropods.
    e. vibrios.

28. Which of these is a type of food poisoning?

    a. Pertussis
    b. Salmonellosis
    c. Gangrene
    d. Chlamydiae
    e. Typhus

29. Which of these statements best describes spores?

    a. They respond to disinfectants.
    b. They are a form of virus.
    c. They are spread through flea bites.
    d. They are smaller than viruses.
    e. They are destroyed through autoclaving.

30. A bull's-eye–shaped rash is one of the most significant symptoms to identify:

    a. Lyme disease.
    b. trachoma.
    c. salmonellosis.
    d. pertussis.
    e. botulism.

31. Which of these diseases is not caused by bacteria?

    a. Strep throat
    b. Scarlet fever
    c. Pneumonia
    d. *Staphylococcus* skin infection
    e. Athlete's foot

32. Tinea capitis is:

    a. nail fungus.
    b. ringworm of the body.
    c. ringworm of the scalp.
    d. athlete's foot.
    e. thrush.

33. Hepatitis, rabies, and polio are diseases caused by:

    a. bacteria.
    b. fungus.
    c. virus.
    d. spirochetes.
    e. Protozoa.

34. What is the common name for the disease pertussis?

    a. Gangrene
    b. Whooping cough
    c. Athlete's foot
    d. Tick-bite disease
    e. Food poisoning

35. Anthrax is caused by:

    a. bacteria.
    b. fungus.
    c. helminths.
    d. Protozoa.
    e. parasites.

36. What organism infects a human from eating uncooked infected beef or pork?

    a. Fluke
    b. Tapeworm
    c. Arthropod
    d. Trichomonas
    e. Rickettsia

37. Which of these is a true statement regarding syphilis?

    a. It is caused from a tick bite.
    b. It is transmitted by eating raw or undercooked meat or fish.
    c. It affects the respiratory tract.
    d. It is caused by a virus.
    e. It is sexually transmitted.

38. Which of these is a bacillus that produces gas in dead tissue?

    a. Tetanus
    b. Tuberculosis
    c. Salmonellosis
    d. Gangrene
    e. Lyme disease

39. Which of these is caused by streptococci?

    a. Botulism
    b. Athlete's foot
    c. Scarlet fever
    d. Syphilis
    e. Typhus

40. Thrush is caused from:

    a. bacteria.
    b. spores.
    c. fungus.
    d. helminths.
    e. Protozoa.

41. Which of these is not recommended as a way to avoid athlete's foot?

    a. Walk barefoot as much as possible to keep your feet dry.
    b. Do not share shoes with others.
    c. Use antifungal powder between your toes.
    d. Change socks frequently.
    e. Wear water shoes in a public shower or locker room.

42. Which of these cause HIV and hepatitis?

    a. Cocci
    b. Virus
    c. Bacilli
    d. Spore
    e. Protozoa

43. Trichomonas are typically found in the:

    a. intestines.
    b. ears.
    c. nose.
    d. throat.
    e. vaginal canal.

44. What condition is caused by Protozoa?

    a. Rabies
    b. Pneumonia
    c. Botulism
    d. Malaria
    e. Polio

45. Tinea unguium is:

    a. nail fungus.
    b. ringworm of the body.
    c. yeast in the mouth.
    d. fungus of the scalp.
    e. thrush.

46. Where are pinworms typically found in the body?

    a. Mouth
    b. Lungs
    c. Rectum
    d. Stomach
    e. Blood vessels

47. Which of these is not an arthropod?

    a. Lice
    b. Spider
    c. Mosquito
    d. Tapeworm
    e. Wasp

48. Which methods of specimen collection is done by the physician?

   a. Venipuncture
   b. Throat swab
   c. Midstream clean-catch urine
   d. Centesis
   e. Wound swab

49. When microbiology tests are performed in the medical office, which of these tasks is not the responsibility of the medical assistant?

   a. Specimen collection
   b. Assisting the physician
   c. Identifying organisms under the microscope
   d. Following standard precautions and safety guidelines
   e. Maintaining asepsis technique

50. Which of these statements is accurate technique when preparing a wet mount?

   a. Allow the fluid to dry on the slide before viewing it.
   b. The slide is viewed under the microscope within 30 minutes.
   c. Wet mounts are only performed on vaginal secretions.
   d. Epithelial cells are not visible in the wet mount.
   e. A wet mount is sent to an outside reference lab for analysis.

51. Which of these represents a gram-positive bacteria?

   a. Entamoeba
   b. Giardia
   c. Trichomonas
   d. E. coli
   e. Staphylococci

BRIEF EXPLANATIONS

52. Explain the difference between aerobic and anaerobic bacteria.

53. What are four (4) basic things necessary for bacteria to grow and survive?

54. Explain the difference in the appearance of diplococci, streptococci, and staphylococci.

_____

_____

_____

_____

55. List two (2) main types of food poisoning and two (2) ways to avoid them.

_____

_____

_____

_____

56. Describe spores, and how they are destroyed.

_____

_____

_____

_____

WHAT DO YOU DO?

57. Read the following scenario and respond to the questions with a short answer.

Steve Zimmerman is a 36-year-old patient who recently returned from business travel to Mexico City. He has not felt well since he returned home to Chicago. He states that he spent a lot of time outdoors sightseeing and got a few mosquito bites. His symptoms include fever, a generalized rash, joint pain, and red eyes. The physician suspects that he has the Zika virus. He orders a CBC and asks the patient to take ibuprofen and rest. The physician instructs the patient to take time off work and return to the office in 3 days for follow-up.

a. As the medical assistant is drawing the patient's blood, he asks her how he got this virus. How would you explain the transmission of the virus?

_____

_____

_____

_____

b. He asks the medical assistant why the physician did not order an antibiotic for this condition. What is your response?

_____

_____

_____

_____

PATIENT EDUCATION

58. Write a short narrative script that you can use to provide patient education about how to stop the spread of disease through good hand hygiene. How does this practice stop the transmission of bacteria?

_____

_____

_____

_____

INTERNET RESEARCH

Visit the Center for Disease Control and Prevention Web site at www.cdc.gov and research foodborne outbreaks. Gather information about one recent outbreak and the investigation that took place. Cite where the outbreak happened, the date(s), what food was involved, and how the outbreak affected the public. What was the outcome of the outbreak? Were any individuals seriously harmed or died from this outbreak?

_____

_____

_____

_____

_____

_____

_____

Procedure 29-1 | Collecting a Specimen for Throat Culture

Name: _____ Date: _____ Time: _____ Grade: _____

Equipment: Tongue blade, sterile specimen container and swab, gloves, a commercial throat culture kit (for testing in the office), laboratory request form, and a biohazard container (for transport to the lab)

Performance Requirement: Student will perform this skill with ____% accuracy not to exceed _____ minutes. (Instructor will determine the point value for each step, % accuracy, and minutes required.)

Performance Checklist

Point Value	Performance Points Earned	Procedure Steps
		1. Wash your hands and put on gloves.
		2. Greet and identify the patient. Explain the procedure.
		3. Ask the patient to sit so a light source is directed at his throat.
		4. Remove the sterile swab from its container.
		5. Ask the patient to say "ahhh" as you press on the midpoint of the tongue with the tongue depressor.
		6. Swab the membranes suspected to be infected. Avoid touching any other areas or structures in the mouth, tongue, or lips with the swab.
		7. Keep holding the tongue depressor in place while removing the swab from your patient's mouth.
		8. Follow the directions on the specimen container for transferring the swab or processing the specimen in the office.
		9. Dispose of supplies and equipment in a biohazard waste container. Remove your gloves and wash your hands.
		10. If sending to a reference lab, prepare the specimen for transport with the lab requisition form.
		11. Document the procedure.

| Procedure 29-1 | Collecting a Specimen for Throat Culture (*Continued*) |

CALCULATION

Total Points Possible: _____

Total Points Earned: _____

Points Earned/Points Possible = _____%

Student completion time (minutes): _____

PASS   FAIL   COMMENTS:

_____

Student's signature _____   Date _____

Instructor's signature _____   Date _____

Procedure 29-2 | Collecting a Sputum Specimen

Name: _____ **Date:** _____ **Time:** _____ **Grade:** _____

Equipment: Labeled sterile specimen container, gloves, laboratory request form, and a biohazard transport container.

Performance Requirement: Student will perform this skill with _____% accuracy not to exceed _____ minutes. (Instructor will determine the point value for each step, % accuracy, and minutes required.)

Performance Checklist

Point Value	Performance Points Earned	Procedure Steps
		1. Wash your hands and put on gloves.
		2. Greet and identify the patient. Explain the procedure. Write the patient's name on a label and put the label on the outside of the container.
		3. Ask the patient to cough deeply. Tell the patient to use the abdominal muscles to bring secretions up from the lungs.
		4. Ask the patient to expectorate directly into the container. Caution him or her not to touch the inside of the container or the specimen becomes contaminated. 5 to 10 mL of sputum is required for most tests.
		5. Handle the specimen container according to standard precautions. Cap the container right away and put it into a transport container marked biohazard.
		6. Fill out the proper laboratory requisition slip.
		7. Care for and dispose of your equipment and supplies. Clean your work area. Then, you can remove your gloves and wash your hands.
		8. Send the specimen to the laboratory immediately.
		9. Document the procedure.

CALCULATION

Total Points Possible: _____

Total Points Earned: _____

Points Earned/Points Possible = _____%

Student completion time (minutes): _____

PASS   FAIL   COMMENTS:

_____

Student's signature _____ Date _____

Instructor's signature _____ Date _____

Procedure 29-3 | Collecting a Stool Specimen

Name: _____ Date: _____ Time: _____ Grade: _____

Equipment: Stool specimen container (for ova and parasite testing), an occult blood test kit (for occult blood testing), and wooden spatulas or tongue blades.

Performance Requirement: Student will perform this skill with ____% accuracy not to exceed _____ minutes. (Instructor will determine the point value for each step, % accuracy, and minutes required.)

Performance Checklist

Point Value	Performance Points Earned	Procedure Steps
		1. Label the container or test kit with the patient's name.
		2. Wash your hands.
		3. Greet and identify the patient. Explain the procedure. Explain any dietary, medication, or other restrictions necessary for the collection.
		4. When collecting a specimen for ova and parasites, tell the patient to collect a small amount of the first and last portion of the stool using the wooden spatula and to place the specimen in the container. Caution the patient not to contaminate the specimen with urine.
		5. When collecting a specimen for occult blood, suggest that the patient obtain the sample from the toilet paper he or she uses to wipe after defecating. Tell the patient to use a wooden spatula to collect the sample. Tell the patient to smear a small amount of the sample from the spatula onto the slide windows.
		6. After the patient returns the stool sample, store the specimen as directed. If instructing the patient to take the specimen directly to a laboratory, give the patient a completed laboratory requisition form.
		7. Document the date and time of the procedure as well as the instructions given to the patient, including the routing procedure.

(Continued)

Procedure 29-3 Collecting a Stool Specimen (*Continued*)

CALCULATION

Total Points Possible: _____

Total Points Earned: _____

Points Earned/Points Possible = _____%

Student completion time (minutes): _____

PASS   FAIL   COMMENTS:

_____

Student's signature _____   Date _____

Instructor's signature _____   Date _____

Procedure 29-4 Testing a Stool Specimen for Occult Blood

Name: _____ Date: _____ Time: _____ Grade: _____

Equipment: Gloves, patient's labeled specimen pack, and developer (or reagent drops).

Performance Requirement: Student will perform this skill with _____% accuracy not to exceed _____ minutes. (Instructor will determine the point value for each step, % accuracy, and minutes required.)

Performance Checklist

Point Value	Performance Points Earned	Procedure Steps
		1. Wash your hands and put on gloves.
		2. Open the test window on the back of the pack. Then, put a drop of the developer or testing reagent on each window according to the manufacturer's directions.
		3. Read the color change within the time specified by the directions. The time is usually 60 seconds.
		4. Put a drop of developer (as directed) on the control monitor section or window of the pack. Take note whether the quality control results are positive or negative, as appropriate.
		5. Use proper procedures to dispose of the test pack and gloves. Wash your hands.
		6. Record the procedure and results.

CALCULATION

Total Points Possible: _____

Total Points Earned: _____

Points Earned/Points Possible = _____%

Student completion time (minutes): _____

PASS   FAIL   COMMENTS:

_____

Student's signature _____ Date _____

Instructor's signature _____ Date _____

Procedure 29-5   Preparing a Wet Mount Slide

Name: _____ **Date:** _____ **Time:** _____ **Grade:** _____

Equipment: Specimen, gloves, microscope slide, sterile saline or 10% potassium hydroxide (**KOH**), coverslip, petroleum jelly, microscope, and pencil or diamond-tipped pen.

Performance Requirement: Student will perform this skill with ____% accuracy not to exceed _____ minutes. (Instructor will determine the point value for each step, % accuracy, and minutes required.)

Performance Checklist

Point Value	Performance Points Earned	Procedure Steps
		1. Wash your hands and put on gloves.
		2. Label the frosted edge of the slide with the patient's name and the date using a pencil or diamond-tipped pen.
		3. Put a drop of the specimen on a glass slide with sterile saline or 10% potassium hydroxide (KOH).
		4. Use a wooden applicator stick to coat the rim of a coverslip with petroleum jelly or spread a thin layer of petroleum jelly on the heal of your gloved hand and then scrape the edges of the coverslip on it to transfer a thin line to each edge. Change the glove before the next step if you use this method.
		5. Put the coverslip over the specimen to keep it from evaporating.
		6. Examine the slide with a microscope using the 40-power objective lens with diminished light.
		7. The physician will examine and read the slide for findings. Microscopic examination is not CLIA-waived testing for medical assistants.
		8. When the physician has completed examining the slide, discard the slide in a biohazard container.
		9. Remove gloves and wash hands.

CALCULATION

Total Points Possible: _____

Total Points Earned: _____

Points Earned/Points Possible = _____%

Student completion time (minutes): _____

PASS   FAIL   COMMENTS:

_____

Student's signature _____ Date _____

Instructor's signature _____ Date _____